Pregnancy

How to Maintain a Healthy Weight Gain during Pregnancy

(How to Eat Well and Maintain Healthy Weight for Mother and Baby)

Nathan Madera

Published By **George Denver**

Nathan Madera

*Pregnancy: How to Maintain a Healthy Weight
Gain during Pregnancy (How to Eat Well and
Maintain Healthy Weight for Mother and Baby)*

ISBN   978-1-7752967-5-1

Legal & Disclaimer

Table Of Contents

Chapter 1: Preparing For Conception

Creating a Healthy Foundation

What if the method of becoming pregnant wasn't as difficult because it seems? When women have a records of the manner their own our bodies feature, they may be capable of clearly conceive, which a lucky scenario is. Furthermore, there are various low-fee and coffee-tech life-style modifications that can assist a female in turning into more wholesome and, probably, developing her opportunities of turning into pregnant.

To start, permit's bypass over the device of concept.

There are some factors which can be required as a manner to get pregnant. To begin, you could want an egg that has reached adulthood and has been launched at some stage in the ovulation way, which takes place as fast as constant with month. Cervical mucus of a immoderate great is likewise required because it not best aids sperm which is probably deposited within the vagina all through sexual hobby to live on, however it furthermore assists them in journeying up the vagina thru the cervix to the component in which they may be part of up with the sperm within the fallopian tube for principle.

The entice is that wonderful cervical mucus, that is often referred to as "egg white cervical mucus" (EWCM) due to the truth that egg whites are a totally accurate description of what it looks as if, is usually best generated within the path of the fertile window of a woman's cycle, that is the duration of her cycle whilst she is able to conceive. When a female is fertile, her window of possibility regularly begins 3 to 5 days in advance than she ovulates and maintains for one to two days after she ovulates. Again, ovulation refers to the gadget wherein one mature egg is released through one of the girl's ovaries. This egg will handiest live on for twelve to twenty-4 hours if it isn't always fertilized via sperm.

Given those worries, a woman's viable window lasts up to round 7 days every menstrual cycle, if you begin counting with the emergence of EWCM 3-five days earlier than ovulation and save you counting forty eight hours afterwards (irrespective of the reality that relying on your man or woman cycle, it would final longer or shorter than that). Outside of your reproductive window, concept can't get up. Contrary to what many humans anticipate, the variety of days every cycle that a lady also can conceive is certainly pretty confined, specially if she has extended or peculiar durations.

The precise statistics, however, is that a pair may also additionally dramatically improve their opportunities of conceiving if they purpose the woman's reproductive window for acts of sexual intercourse. Some specialists urge that couples have intercourse every other day sooner or later of the fertile window (in vicinity of each day) for maximal sperm fitness.

That's turning into pregnant at its most crucial. All of the troubleshooting round infertility with fertility awareness techniques (FAMs) of natural own family planning (NFP) and Restorative Reproductive Medicine (RRM), as NaProTechnology does, basically explores the motives why one or greater of these essential components preferred for idea is lacking or malfunctioning.

Five techniques to reinforce your opportunities of conceiving

1. Eat a healthful healthy dietweight-reduction plan and pursue a balanced manner of lifestyles

Thankfully, there are low-tech way of lifestyles adjustments you may do in recent times to beautify your great fitness, and ideally your possibilities of conceiving. You can decrease your usage of alcohol, coffee, and chocolates, and quit smoking. Moderate aerobic hobby three-4 instances consistent with week is an nearly unanimous idea for ladies looking to gain pregnant.

Eating a weight loss program low in processed elements and wealthy of dark, leafy vegetables and colorful end result and veggies corresponds with more trendy health. Beyond that massive tenet, a few studies shows that what you eat ought to in all likelihood definitely assist balance your hormone ranges and increase your possibilities of conceiving. If it intrigues you, test into seed cycling or these trusted dietary supplements.

2. Make tremendous your capsules aren't adversely influencing your fertility

Additionally, you may have a examine if any of your frequently scheduled prescriptions intrude with cervical mucus manufacturing, as happens with sure antidepressants, epilepsy meds, antihistamines, and allergic reaction capsules Talk collectively along with your health practitioner about one in every of a type selections that may match your necessities at the identical time as looking to conceive.

3. Seek therapy for hormonal troubles

Keep in thoughts, but, that during case you've got been previously on a form of hormonal beginning control, your frame may moreover need many cycles to reset and obtain the right hormone levels critical to come to be (and continue to be) pregnant. Note, however, that if you bought on the pill to "regulate" your cycle, you have to expect that the semblance of "law" will give up with the capsules, thinking about delivery manage is simply a band-aid for hormonal imbalances and not a treatment. If your shipping manage emerge as formerly disguising a hormonal imbalance and it returns, you can need to first are looking for remedy from a restorative reproductive care professional so that you can grow to be pregnant truly.

four. Get tested for sexually transmitted ailments (STIs)

Getting tested for STIs (and treated, if applicable) is straight forward, and an easy check-off on the "activities to conceive" listing, as first-class STIs immediately harm your possibilities of conceiving.

5. Manage strain

Stress manage may be very crucial for girls seeking to conceive without a doubt, normally because of the truth a always physical or emotionally burdened individual's body will react thru pumping out the pressure hormone cortisol. While the precise mechanisms aren't absolutely recognized, we do realize that once the frame is consistently in overdrive liberating cortisol, in the long run progesterone manufacturing and ovulation are notably impacted. Low progesterone degrees can also impair every your capability to become pregnant and to stay pregnant. Managing your pressure, then, through self-care, mindfulness, guided meditation, prayer, and remedy, can also additionally definitely make a distinction in your choice to conceive. There is also an first-rate beneficial resource referred to as Organic Conceptions, that would help couples within the route of superior mental health on their travels within the route of concept.

The unmarried maximum vital factor you can do to come to be pregnant is...

Exercising, consuming healthy, and proscribing your caffeine intake are all useful way of life enhancements to adopt in case you're seeking out to conceive. The single maximum massive component you may do to reinforce your possibilities of becoming pregnant, but, is to check a fertility attention method (FAM) from a expert trainer (the professional instructor element is important, no longer trivial).

Why need to you examine a FAM even if you're not tremendous you need to adopt entire attempting out and diagnostic workups? The single maximum critical motive to research a FAM in case you're searching for to conceive clearly is that you can learn how to select out your body's personal symptoms and symptoms of fertility, mainly the adjustments in consistency, colour, and amount of cervical mucus that correlate with a cyclical shift from infertility (maximum of the cycle) to fertility (the fertile window). These days, there's an effective, proof-based totally definitely FAM for nearly every way of life, which include swing shift human beings, people with unpredictable sleep-wake cycles, and so on.

That's not all you'll get from studying a FAM, but. Learning to tune your cycle by using writing down on paper (or setting into an app) the custom designed, seen facts points like cervical mucus and temperature variations that your body presents you on a each day foundation, isn't first-class some issue you do at the same time as you're scared that some element's incorrect. Learning to chart your cycle is beneficial for each girl, irrespective of whether or not you're currently attempting to find to conceive or no longer, due to the fact reproductive fitness is an indicator of tremendous health inside the body, essential a few to even call it "the 5th essential signal." You can monitor your heart health thru your

Apple iWatch, and you could show your reproductive fitness via your cycle charting.

Increasing your frame literacy can also lead you to reveal grace to yourself while you're managing a large artwork reduce-off date clearly as "that point of the month" is coming, to sense more cushty on your non-public pores and skin, and to art work collectively together with your frame in preference to in the direction of it.

If required, you could make use of that records to work with a expert healthcare expert to troubleshoot concerns like PMS, bizarre bleeding, weird intervals, and, certain, infertility, which isn't a number one evaluation itself, however is instead a demonstration of some trouble else being incorrect. But you don't need to wait until some aspect is inaccurate to are available touch collectively with your body by using way of studying a FAM.

Section

- Lifestyle Choices and Their Impact

At our sanatorium, we frequently get requested the same question: "What can I do to enhance my probabilities of conceiving without a doubt?" It's a question we adore to pay interest because it suggests that our patients are invested of their reproductive health. And the answer is that the cornerstone of a strong being pregnant starts with a healthy basis.

Many human beings have been made to assume that becoming pregnant is simple and can display up every time we choice. While this will be real for a few ladies of their 20s, the reality is that fertility falls as we age. Extra interest and interest may be required to decorate health so a a success pregnancy is feasible.

Currently, "...greater people are delaying having youngsters till their overdue 30s or 40s. As you age, so do your ovaries and the eggs inner them. You cannot see or experience these modifications, and that they show up quicker than you can expect. A girl's excessive reproductive years are a number of the past due young adults and late 20s. By age 30, the capability to end up pregnant begins offevolved to wane and it takes vicinity quicker till you reach your mid-30s. By forty five, fertility has fallen so extensively that becoming pregnant absolutely isn't always going." (ACOG FAQ)

As increasing couples favor to delay having a infant into their 30s and 40s, it's important to emphasise life-style picks that promote a robust basis for concept and a a fulfillment being pregnant. Unfortunately, the reality is that hundreds folks in this age institution have stressful existence, regularly consuming on the bypass, getting insufficient sleep with era in our beds, and being exposed to dangerous chemicals.

These regular alternatives also can make contributions to a "confused frame" kingdom, on the equal time because the sympathetic (fight or flight) nerve device prevails, and the reproductive gadget can be damaged, crucial to decrease fertility.

What is Fight (Sympathetic) Mode?

The sympathetic concerned device is chargeable for the frame's reaction to a perceived risk, normally referred to as the "fight or flight" reaction. When engaged, this tool can also prompt a state of heightened pressure, similar to the experience of being in a heated fight or receiving a surprising surprise or terror. Prolonged publicity to this condition of heightened strain may additionally increase to continual strain, that may have detrimental influences on each our physical and highbrow fitness.

Our our our bodies respond to the dispute or the imagined fear/pressure in high-quality techniques:

Increase in coronary heart rate, blood pressure, and respiration charge, (panting or shortness of breath)

Focus and attentiveness upward thrust (an excessive amount of),

Our eyes get broader (dilated)

Digestion shuts down (constipation)

The thoughts races (insomnia), tough to calm down

No interest in intercourse.

A sudden surge of hormones will increase the body's attentiveness delivering more blood to the muscle tissues promotes perspiration

Activate goose bumps

The combat (sympathetic) mode is a herbal healthful reaction whilst it's miles episodic (brief time period). It is a style that is supposed to be entirely for survival, actually stay or death. When this pattern turns into the norm day over day and 12 months over 12 months, our bodily structures begin to push back, in massive part from of tiredness, within the fertility situation – we do no longer grow to be pregnant in this mode.

After all, you'll now not force a vehicle the fastest it could skip for three years immediately...the automobile has to stop and relaxation for servicing, petrol, additives, washing and clean oil to hold this rapid driving.

What is Flight (Parasympathetic) Mode

The parasympathetic worried device is chargeable for the body's rest and digests reaction even as the frame is in a cushty or resting condition. This mechanism efficaciously reverses the consequences of the sympathetic nervous device after a length of pressure.

When engaged, the parasympathetic nervous device slows down breathing and coronary heart price and aids digestion. By putting in place a rustic of rest and serenity, the parasympathetic irritating gadget can also help lower stress tiers and increase modern-day nicely-being.

In the parasympathetic mode:

Our heart price and respiratory prices slow down

Blood strain is decreased

Digestion is optimized with the resource of the use of extended digestive enzymes

The bronchial tubes constrict – pass lower again to regular

Muscles loosen up all all through the body

When we advantage a degree of relaxation, our our our bodies engage their inherent healing, healing, and cleansing methods. Being inside the parasympathetic vicinity greater frequently can also additionally promote extra fitness and beautify the possibility of having pregnant. However, our contemporary life are the alternative of what our our our bodies are constructed for.

Instead of dwelling inside the parasympathetic location with occasional sympathetic episodes, we generally generally tend to live inside the sympathetic location, with the parasympathetic United States of America being an first rate. This also can additionally result in the choice to turn to lousy behaviors together with eating junk meals, consuming, and being sedentary in the front of the TV as a technique of comforting ourselves.

At any age we can also additionally begin be aware about what our body's require to flourish. It is important to differentiate the combat (sympathetic mode) strolling swiftly from the aggressor or flight (parasympathetic mode) the rest, digest, art work life balance. Nurturing the relaxation and digest facet and developing techniques to feel pride gives a platform to assist the frame say "positive" to principle.

Timing:

The handiest way to a wholesome being pregnant is to permit for a time of three-6 months to boom a solid and healthy foundation. During this era, it's recommended to look an OB/Gyn for a complete take a look at-up and bloodwork. Then discover Chinese Medicine to help stability hormones and optimize menstrual cycles to assure strong and everyday ovulation, and lessen signs and symptoms of PMS. This is specially critical for girls who have been the usage of start manipulate for prolonged intervals.

First stuff First:

Schedule a check-up with your OB/Gyn and notify them about your aspirations to conceive. During the appointment, request routine blood art work along with a whole blood chemistry (CBC), thyroid, weight loss plan D, fasting glucose, and A1C, in addition to a PAP.

These modern tests also can display small abnormalities that might have an impact to your pregnancy and may be treated earlier. Skipping this step would possibly result in dropping out on vital statistics, and wearing out those workups can regularly avoid miscarriage. This is an tremendous starting area.

Feed your Body:

Although no longer a glamorous issue, it's miles vitally vital to do not forget ingesting a healthful food plan. .A terrible weight-reduction plan locations your body beneath even greater strain as it needs to artwork tougher to assimilate chemicals, poisons, and occasional-first-rate meals, which consumes a extremely good amount of electricity.

This power need to preferably cross within the route of fuelling your hormones favorably. Opting to pay attention on limiting sugar intake, consuming masses of veggies, a few surrender result, nuts, and oils – a severa sort of meals – will dramatically decorate your possibilities of conceiving and positioned your frame decrease once more into balance. In certain situations, this by myself can also lead to a a hit being pregnant!

Last:

Addressing in which the primary stresses are in existence and taking efforts to lessen them locations us right away in the parasympathetic mode (relaxation and relax).

Studies have indicated that acupuncture might also moreover set off the parasympathetic nerve device, this is responsible for the frame's rest response. By activating the parasympathetic mode with acupuncture, patients may also enjoy decrease stress, extended sleep, and higher not unusual health.

Acupuncture and natural treatment additionally work carefully with the Vagus nerve it clearly is part of the parasympathetic (rest, relax) gadget.

The great route to idea is to increase a amazing foundation, the preliminary building stones is probably the hardest.

Chapter 2: Navigating the Trimesters

From First Trimester Challenges to Third Trimester Preparations

An unborn little one spends more or a great deal much less 38 weeks within the womb, but the not unusual length of being pregnant (gestation) is seemed as forty weeks.

This is because of the fact pregnancy is counted from the first day of the woman's final menstruation, no longer the day of thought, which typically happens 2 weeks later.

Pregnancy is normally split into 3 durations called trimesters of spherical three months each :

first trimester from concept to twelve weeks

second trimesterthirteen to 27 weeks

1/three trimester28 to 40 weeks.

Length of being pregnant also can variety among girls — toddlers are deemed 'whole time period' if they may be born someplace between 37-42 weeks.

First trimester of pregnancyconcept to twelve weeks

Symptoms and signs of early pregnancy encompass:

neglected periods

nausea and vomiting (morning sickness)

breast modifications

tiredness

common urination.

If you're experiencing any of those symptoms and believe you'll be pregnant, it's miles a first-rate idea to take a being pregnant test.

If you failed to anticipate to get pregnant, it's miles important to have a being pregnant take a look at as quickly as you could. The faster a being pregnant is showed, the sooner you can get treatment, and the greater options may be open to you.

During the primary trimester, miscarriage is common. Around 1 in 4 pregnancies result in miscarriage. Most spontaneous miscarriages (75 to eighty consistent with cent) arise within the first 12 weeks. Many miscarriages are unreported or go unrecognised because of the truth they stand up extraordinarily early in being pregnant.

Conception

The 2d of concept takes vicinity on the same time as the girl's ovum (egg) is fertilised via the person's sperm. The gender and hereditary capabilities are determined in that 2d.

Pregnancy week 1

This first week is definitely your menstrual cycle. Because your predicted begin or due date (EDD or EDB) is decided from the primary day of your very last duration, this week counts as part of your forty-week being pregnant, even in case your infant hasn't been created however. If you understand the day of your final duration, you can use a gestation calculator to decide your due date.

Pregnancy week 2

Fertilisation of your egg with the aid of way of using the sperm (called idea) will take place on the perception of this week.

Pregnancy week three

Thirty hours after idea, the cell breaks into . Three days later, the cell (zygote) splits into 16 cells. After more days, the zygote has traveled from the fallopian tube to the uterus (womb). Seven days after perception, the zygote burrows itself into the fat uterine lining (endometrium). The zygote is now referred to as a blastocyst.

Pregnancy week four

The developing toddler is tinier than a grain of rice. The swiftly dividing cells are in the method of developing the severa physical systems, such as the digestive system.

Pregnancy week 5

The developing neural tube will in the long run emerge as the extensive worried machine (mind and spinal cord).

Pregnancy week 6

The infant is now known as an embryo. It is greater or much less three mm in period. By this time, it's miles secreting unique hormones that save you the mom from having a menstrual length.

Pregnancy week 7

The coronary heart is pounding. The embryo has mounted its placenta and amniotic sac. The placenta is burrowing into the uterine wall to get oxygen and vitamins from the mother's move.

Pregnancy week 8

The embryo is now kind of 1.Three cm in length. The swiftly growing spinal wire looks as if a tail. The head is excessively big.

Pregnancy week nine

The eyes, lips and tongue are growing. The small muscles enable the embryo to begin shifting round. Blood cells are being generated through the use of the embryo's liver.

Pregnancy week 10

The embryo is now known as a fetus and is extra or a lot much less 2.Five cm in length. All of the body organs are advanced. The fingers and feet, which in advance seemed like nubs or paddles, in the meanwhile are growing fingers and ft. The mind is energetic and has thoughts waves.

Pregnancy week eleven

Teeth are growing within the gums. The small coronary coronary heart is developing similarly.

Pregnancy week 12

The hands and ft are identifiable, but though effective collectively with webs of pores and pores and pores and skin. The first trimester mixture screening check (maternal blood check + ultrasound of little one) may be carried out round this era. This check examines for trisomy 18 (Edward syndrome) and trisomy 21 (Down syndrome).

Second trimester of being pregnant — 13 weeks to 27 weeks

The 2nd trimester of being pregnant commonly begins round weeks 13 and 14. During this era, maximum women find out that morning contamination eases and that they've greater power.

Your being pregnant can be critical and you could have received some weight. Steady weight boom in a few unspecified time in the destiny of being pregnant is regular and beneficial for the health of you and your child. However, it's far similarly important not to gather an excessive amount of weight by using adopting a balanced food regimen and exercising often.

Gestational diabetes is commonly recognized around weeks 24 to twenty-8 of being pregnant, however it could occur quicker.

Pregnancy week 13

The fetus can swim round pretty aggressively. It is currently more than 7 centimeters in duration.

Pregnancy week 14

The eyelids are fused over the without a doubt grown eyes. The toddler can now mutely cry, because it has vocal chords. It may even start sucking its thumb. The hands and feet are sprouting nails.

Pregnancy week sixteen

The fetus is form of 14 cm in length. Eyelashes and eyebrows have fashioned, and the tongue has taste buds. The 2d trimester maternal serum screening may be supplied proper now if the number one trimester check have emerge as no longer executed (see week 12).

Pregnancy weeks 18-20

An ultrasound can be supplied. This prenatal morphology test is to show for structural abnormalities, vicinity of placenta and multiple pregnancies. Interestingly, hiccoughs in the fetus may frequently be decided.

Pregnancy week 20

The fetus is type of 21 cm in length. Its ears are certainly running and it could pay interest muted noises from the outer global. The palms have prints. The genitals may additionally moreover now be differentiated the use of an ultrasound take a look at.

Pregnancy week 24

The fetus is greater or plenty much less 33 cm in duration. The fused eyelids now break up into better and reduce lids, permitting the trendy toddler to open and near its eyes. The pores and skin is included in excellent hair (lanugo) and covered thru a layer of waxy secretion (vernix). The little one creates respiration motions with its lungs.

Third trimester of pregnancy — 28 weeks to 40 weeks

During the zero.33 trimester your infant is developing rapid and you may revel in more exhausted. You may be conscious changes on your frame as your child grows. In the later weeks your toddler will frequently descend all the way all the way down to has interaction (or 'drop') into your pelvis to put together for transport.

It isn't unusual to experience anxious, undergo again ache, dyspnea and sleep troubles as difficult paintings methods. Although preeclampsia may additionally rise up at any 2nd at a few level inside the second one half of being pregnant, there can be a bigger chance of it developing at some stage in this era.

Pregnancy week 28

Your teenager now weighs spherical 1 kg (1,000 g) or 2 lb 2oz (2 pounds, 2 oz..) and measures approximately 25 cm (10 inches) from crown to rump. The crown-to-toe duration is more or less 37 cm. The growing frame has caught up with the large head and the little one now appears extra in percent.

Pregnancy week 32

The newborn spends a super deal of its time napping. Its motions are strong and synchronized. It has probable obtained the 'head down' posture via now, in steering for shipping.

Pregnancy week 36

The infant is form of forty six centimeters in period. It has probably tucked its head into its mother's pelvis, making ready for transport. If it is born nowadays, its possibilities for survival are tremendous. Development of the lungs is rapid in the route of the subsequent numerous weeks.

Pregnancy week 40

The child is form of fifty one cm in duration and prepared to be birthed. It is uncertain precisely what triggers the commencement of labour. It is most likely a mixture of physical, hormonal and emotional interactions most of the mother and toddler.

- Celebrating Milestones and Managing Changes

If you've been dreaming of parenting, finding out you're pregnant should probably enjoy unreal. As your pregnancy continues, aches and pains may additionally need to placed a bit of a damper for your enthusiasm, however with each milestone the satisfaction of being closer and toward seeing your infant may also strike domestic.

We understand what you're questioning: What are those milestones and while do they get up?

Every being pregnant is first-rate and each mother may also have their private specific reminiscences, however we've superior a listing of some of our favorite being pregnant milestones you may encounter. We want you'll go through in mind the ones unique activities to pause and scent the pregnant plant life.

Early pregnancy milestones

Experiencing initial pregnancy symptoms

For many girls, lacking their length is the number one indicator that they may be pregnant. However, a few mothers-to-be endure morning contamination pretty early on or face some considerable mood adjustments.

While feeling ill and being distinctly emotional won't appear to be a few component to have an awesome time, in case you've been trying to have a little one, the ones preliminary being pregnant signs may be motive for exceptional pride.

Pregnancy Symptoms: 10 Early Signs That You May Be Pregnant

Getting a fantastic pregnancy check

Once you trust it's viable you'll be pregnant, maximum human beings want to recognize for high quality proper away right now! Home being pregnant checks rely upon growing hCG levels in your urine to discover if you may be pregnant.

How early for your being pregnant you could gather dependable check outcomes varies at the individual being pregnant check, but the week following your lacking period is a commonplace time for hCG tiers to be excessive sufficient to file excellent.

Having your first prenatal checkup

Many expectant mother and father get their first prenatal checkup about 8 weeks into their pregnancy. After the questions, examination, and blood test, the fact which you're pregnant might also virtually strike home!

Hearing your little one's heartbeat

Vaginal ultrasound may come across a baby's heartbeat as early as five half to six weeks into the pregnancy. Hopefully your medical medical doctor is probably able to choose out up your little one's heartbeat at some level in the preliminary ultrasound, however if it's no longer feasible to pay attention the coronary heart beat, your clinical clinical physician may moreover ask you to return in a week or to attempt yet again.

By weeks 6 and seven, the pulse need to be among 90 and a hundred and ten beats consistent with minute (bpm) and via nine weeks the coronary coronary heart beat need to have climbed to 140 to one hundred and seventy bpm.

Seeing your infant on ultrasound

Depending to your medical records and your doctor's choice, you can get the number one ultrasound from 7 half of to eight weeks into your being pregnant. This early within the being pregnant a transvaginal ultrasound will be done.

Some physicians don't order the primary ultrasound till eleven to 14 weeks but. As your being pregnant advances you're in all likelihood to get an stomach ultrasound.

If you have got got a statistics of miscarriage, fertility problems, or have had a tough pregnancy inside the past, your medical doctor can also furthermore prescribe an early first ultrasound at 6 weeks gestation. This will provide a risk to affirm the fetus' feature and size.

Telling buddies or own family you're looking forward to

While some individuals choose to wait in order that there's a dwindled opportunity of miscarriage, others can't wait to cellular cellphone everybody in the prolonged circle of relatives with the completely glad facts a child is at the manner right away after the effective pregnancy test.

There isn't always any right or incorrect in phrases of the question of whilst to inform. A

2008 studies indicated that when 6 weeks, the possibility of miscarriage following a tested heartbeat is tons a good deal less than 10 percent.

There also are countless strategies to keep the extremely good statistics for your social community. How you inform others might create for memorable reminiscences!

Buying first infant item

You might not have even been pregnant however whilst you got the primary object for your destiny teen — or you may have delayed buying some thing until the final weeks of your pregnancy.

There are numerous forms of gadgets you could pick to build up, however some thing you select will surely occupy a specific place on your coronary coronary heart and your infant's nursery.

Craving — or warding off! — food

Many ladies enjoy being pregnant cravings and nutritional aversions as early because of the reality the first trimester. These normally rise up within the course of the second one trimester and reduce inside the 0.33 trimester.

While many ladies want goodies, carbohydrates, or salty topics, each pregnancy and lady is particular. Keeping notes of the dreams and aversions you encounter might be a great memory to appearance decrease once more on when you supply begin.

Mid-pregnancy milestones

Reaching the second trimester

The 2d trimester ranges from weeks 13 to 27. Since this is the trimester whilst many girls start to without a doubt enjoy their frame bodily trade, it can be a length while your pregnancy seems exceedingly right.

Reaching the second one trimester can be a motive for pleasure as morning infection and numerous special first trimester symptoms lighten up.

Finding out the sex

There are numerous strategies to discover the intercourse of your teen, and depending at the method you pick upon, you could discover at some of precise stages!

If your being pregnant began through manner of technique of having an embryo implanted, you've possibly mentioned the sex of your toddler while you preserve in mind that before you have got been even pregnant. Alternatively, you may have opted to take a completely each other approach and now not discover the intercourse until after the infant is added!

Ultrasound may additionally moreover can help you discover the sex. Most physicians look at this at some point of an ultrasound performed amongst 18 to 21 weeks, but it could be completed as early as 14 weeks.

Wearing being pregnant apparel

By the time you're many months into your pregnancy, you could study that your body is beginning to regulate enough that your conventional clothing now not feels cushty. Of reality, this could arise masses quicker depending for your frame kind and if that is a 2nd or zero.33 pregnancy.

While adapting on your altered shape can also additionally bring severa emotions, maternity put on is assured to supply a breath of comfort after the tightness of your widespread jeans! This moreover approach you're in fact showing more, and others can also moreover furthermore word your pregnancy.

Feeling toddler flow into

Your kid has been transferring for the reason that save you of the number one trimester, but you probable acquired't experience it until at the earliest 13 weeks. (And that's normally without a doubt if you've been pregnant previously and realize what those tiny flutters are!)

As the second trimester maintains, you're likely to experience more potent and stronger kicks. This might be unpleasant, however moreover immensely encouraging that your youngster continues to be doing nicely.

Having someone else revel in little one bypass

Your companion will frequently be capable of enjoy motion some weeks at the same time as you do. If they're laying their palm on your tummy, they may experience the child wriggling approximately as early as 20 weeks. (As time goes on, they'll also be able to test movement from the out of doors, which may be each extraordinary wonderful second.)

By approximately 25 weeks, your toddler should begin to react to acquainted sounds, and your associate may moreover additionally additionally be capable of cause a few kicks actually via speakme to the child!

End-of-being pregnant milestones

Reaching the zero.33 trimester

Once to procure week 28, you can have amusing reaching the 0.33 trimester. Your teen is probably complete time period through the prevent of week 37, and that's a fantastic success!

Celebrating your little one-to-be

Two terms... child bathe! This collecting might be a awesome event to come back together with all the massive people to your existence. There aren't any hard-and-fast policies on while this celebration want to be held or maybe what it need to look like, so the maximum critical thing is absolutely to revel in this particular time.

However, if situations don't permit for a bath, don't feel such as you've wasted a while to have a good time. Taking images, writing, and in any other case recording your being pregnant is a protracted-lasting way to honor your street to parenting.

Reaching your due date

If you haven't long beyond into difficult paintings by the point your due date comes spherical, you may be equipped to throw within the towel. It would possibly probably experience along with you've been pregnant for all of the time.

It's vital to keep in mind that your due date is an expected shipping date (based totally totally mostly on both the date of your closing length or information from an ultrasound), and your toddler is probably proper right here right away. While 60 percent of pregnant human beings supply on or earlier than their due date, that leaves loads of pregnancies that boom most effective a piece longer.

Feeling exertions start

Whether your hard work starts offevolved with a normal construct-up of contractions, a gush of water at the same time as your amniotic sac breaches, or a planned appointment for induction or a C-segment, it's all part of your character hard work narrative.

The birthing experience is special for each individual (and varies each time you deliver shipping), so you also can experience hundreds of anticipation leading as plenty as the onset of hard paintings. When you find out your tough paintings has commenced out, you can revel in widespread excitement.

Meeting your new toddler

Assuming the entirety goes properly, you're in all likelihood to discover yourself with a small new infant package deal deal deal in your chest inside mins of begin. This might be loads to soak up!

You can also discover yourself sobbing, fatigued, perplexed, or honestly passionately in love. Whatever emotions you experience, you could want a person to lure this on video, so you'll normally have it documented.

Of route the fun is really as robust and overwhelming in case your come across is delayed or now not what you anticipated. Whether you deliver and beginning your toddler yourself, have your first assembly due to surrogacy or adoption, or something your tale unfolds, the on the spot you observe your little one for the primary time is a memorable one.

Takeaway

Pregnancy might not constantly be glamorous; however there may be a few relatively memorable studies alongside the journey to assembly your toddler.

From first kicks to informing your own family and locating out the intercourse, it's important to take a pause and recognize all the tiny milestones alongside the route.

Chapter 3: Physical and Emotional Well-Being

Nutritional Guidance and Exercise Practices

Having a infant is an thrilling time that often pushes girls to undertake better lifestyle alternatives and, if required, purpose closer to a healthful frame weight. Here you'll find out recommendation on how to decorate your food and physical interest conduct at the same time as you're pregnant and after your teen is born.

These recommendations can be beneficial if you're not pregnant however are considering having a child! By making changes these days, you could end up adjusted to new lifestyle patterns. You'll provide your little one the finest feasible begin on existence and be a healthy instance in your circle of relatives for an entire life.

A pregnant girl wanders in the woods with her husband and little daughter.

Being active at the same time as you're pregnant also can assist you have a wholesome pregnancy.

Healthy Weight

Why is gaining a wholesome quantity of weight in some unspecified time inside the future of pregnancy crucial?

Gaining a suitable amount of weight during being pregnant permits your toddler boom to a healthy length But gaining an excessive amount of or too little weight might also motive number one fitness headaches for you and your toddler.

According to specialists External hyperlink, gaining an excessive amount of weight at some stage in being pregnant complements your threat for buying gestational diabetes (diabetes in a few unspecified time within the destiny of being pregnant) and excessive blood strain at some stage in pregnancy. It also will growth your hazard for type 2 diabetes and excessive blood stress later in life. If you're obese or have weight issues at the same time as you grow to be pregnant, your danger for fitness problems may be notably extra. You may additionally moreover be much more likely to have a cesarean phase (C-segment) NIH out of doors hyperlink.

Gaining a wholesome amount of weight lets in you have got were given have been given an simpler being pregnant and delivery. It also can help make it plenty less hard a brilliant manner to pass again to a wholesome weight following beginning. Research well-known that counseled ranges of weight benefit during being pregnant might also reduce the possibilities which you or your teenager can also have weight troubles and weight-associated issues later in life.

How an awful lot weight must I accumulate in some unspecified time in the future of my being pregnant?

How masses weight you have to gather relies upon on your body mass index (BMI) in advance than being pregnant. BMI is a measure of your weight in proportion on your pinnacle. You may moreover use a manner to determine your BMI NIH outside hyperlink online.

The conventional weight-advantage advice beneath is for women having honestly one toddler.

If you1 You ought to accumulate round

Are underweight (BMI much less than 18.Five) 28 to forty kilos

Are at a healthful weight (BMI of 18.Five to 24.Nine) 25 to 35 kilos

Are obese (BMI of 25 to 29.Nine) 15 to 20-5 kilos

Have weight problems (BMI of 30+) 11 to 20 pounds

It's crucial to collect weight very slowly. The conventional misconception which you're "eating for two" isn't accurate. During the primary three months, your youngster is without a doubt the dimensions of a walnut and doesn't require many greater calories. The following pace of weight growth is usually encouraged

1 to 4 kilos fashionable in the first 3 months

2 to four pounds in keeping with month from 4 months until delivery

Talk to your health care professional about how an lousy lot weight benefit is appropriate for you. Work with her or him to growth dreams in your weight benefit. Take into hobby your age, weight, and health. Track your weight at domestic or when you see your health care issuer.

Don't try and shed pounds if you're pregnant. Your little one desires to be uncovered to healthy food and low-calorie drinks (particularly water) to increase efficiently. Some women may furthermore lose a modest little bit of weight during the onset of pregnancy. Speak to your fitness care practitioner if this takes vicinity to you.

Healthy Eating

How a incredible deal ought to I eat and drink?

Consuming healthful food and coffee-calorie liquids, particularly water, and the maximum beneficial quantity of power also assist you to and your infant collect the quality quantity of weight.

How masses meals and what number of electricity you require depends on factors in conjunction with your weight in advance than being pregnant, your age, and the way suddenly you gain weight. If you're at a healthy weight, the Centers for Disease Control and Prevention (CDC) External link says you want no extra energy in your first trimester, approximately 340 greater power a day on your 2nd trimester, and approximately 450 extra energy an afternoon on your 0.33 trimester.1 You additionally may not need extra energy within the direction of the very last weeks of being pregnant.

Check at the side of your health care practitioner about your weight advantage. If you're not gaining the burden you need, he or she also can urge you to take in extra power. If you're gaining an excessive amount of weight, you may want to cut down on power. Each lady's necessities are precise. Your necessities additionally depend on whether or not you've got were given been underweight, overweight, or had weight problems before you've got been pregnant, or if you're having multiple teen.

What forms of food and drink must I devour?

A weight loss plan inside the course of pregnancy consists of nutrient-rich food and beverages. The Dietary Guidelines for Americans, 2020–2025 External hyperlinks advise the ones meals and beverages every day

Give up result and veggies (deliver vitamins and fiber)

Complete grains, along with oatmeal, entire-grain bread, and brown rice (deliver fiber, B nutrients and different required vitamins)

Fats-free or low-fats milk and milk merchandise or nondairy soy, almond, rice, or certainly one of a kind drinks with greater calcium and nutrients D

protein from healthful assets, together with beans and peas, eggs, lean meats, seafood this is low in mercury (as much as 12 oz.. In line with week), and unsalted nuts and seeds, if you may belly them and aren't allergic to them.

A healthy eating plan furthermore reduces salt, solid fat (together with butter, lard, and shortening), and sugar-sweetened beverages and meals.

A display off of sparkling vegetables, beans, fruit, seafood, lean proteins, accurate fats, whole grains, and milk

Fruit, colorful vegetables, legumes, seafood, and coffee-fat dairy are amazing assets of nutrients required at some stage in being pregnant.

Does your eating plan measure up? How are you able to decorate your habits? Try ingesting fruit like berries or a banana with warm or bloodless cereal for morning; a salad with beans or tofu or extraordinary non-meat protein for lunch; and a lean dish of meat, fowl, turkey, or fish with steamed greens for dinner. Think of latest, healthy food and drinks you may try. Write down your thoughts and communicate them together together with your health care practitioner.

A dinner of steamed vegetables and grilled chook breast affords nutrients without too many calories.

What if I'm a vegetarian?

A vegetarian dietary plan within the course of pregnancy can be healthy. Consider the exceptional of your consuming plan and chat on your health care expert to make sure you're receiving sufficient calcium, iron, protein, weight-reduction plan B12, diet regime D, and different critical minerals. Your fitness care expert might also educate you to take nutrients and minerals that will help you satisfy your desires.

Do I honestly have any particular dietary requirements now that I'm pregnant?

Yes. During being pregnant, you want extra nutrients and minerals which include folate, iron, and calcium.

Getting the final amount of folate is extraordinarily important. Folate, a B vitamins moreover called folic acid, can also help save you start abnormalities. Before pregnancy, you need four hundred mcg in step with day from dietary supplements or fortified food, similarly to the folate you purchased manifestly from food and beverages. During being pregnant, you need six hundred mcg. While nursing, you want 500 mcg of folate steady with day.2 Foods rich in folate encompass orange juice, strawberries, spinach, broccoli, beans, fortified breads, and fortified low-sugar breakfast cereals. These elements also can additionally probable deliver 100% of the everyday rate of folic acid everyday with serving.

Most health care specialists encourage women who're pregnant to take a prenatal food regimen each day and eat healthy food, snacks, and drinks. Ask your medical doctor approximately what you should take.

What particular new behaviors may additionally useful beneficial resource my weight benefit?

Pregnancy can also furthermore generate some new meals, beverage, and ingesting issues. Meet the needs of your frame and be more snug with those suggestions. Check together collectively together with your health care practitioner with any problems.

Eat breakfast every day. If you experience sick on your belly within the morning, attempt dry complete-wheat toast or entire-grain crackers at the same time as you first wake up. Eat them even in advance than you get out of bed. Eat the the rest of your breakfast (fruit, oatmeal, heat or cold cereal, or awesome devices) later in the morning.

Eat excessive-fiber food. Eating immoderate-fiber meals, ingesting water, and obtaining normal bodily exercising may moreover assist keep away from constipation. Try to consume whole-grain cereals, brown rice, veggies, give up end result, and legumes.

If you revel in heartburn, eat small meals scattered in some unspecified time in the destiny of the day. Try to devour slowly and keep away from highly spiced and fatty meals (consisting of warm peppers or fried bird). Have beverages amongst meals instead of with meals. Don't lay down rapidly after consuming.

Dish of cooked black beans with bell peppers and brown rice.

High-fiber meals like beans can keep away from constipation in some unspecified time in the future of pregnancy.

What food and drinks need to I avoid?

Certain ingredients and liquids can also damage your baby if you consume them even as you're pregnant. Here's a list of merchandise you need to avoid.

Alcohol Do not consume alcohol, together with wine, beer, or robust liquor.

Caffeine Enjoy decaf espresso or tea, drinks no longer sweetened with sugar, or water with a sprint of juice. Avoid food plan beverages, and restriction drinks with caffeine to much less than two hundred mg in keeping with day—the amount in round 12 ouncesof coffee.Three

Fish that could encompass excessive quantities of mercury (a chemical that might growth in fish and damage an unborn infant) Limit white (albacore) tuna to six ounces constant with week Do not consume king mackerel, marlin, orange roughly, shark, swordfish, or tilefish. To collect the vital nutrients in fish and shellfish, you could devour up to 12 ounces of seafood each week, deciding on from numerous wholesome seafood options External link, which encompass cod, salmon, and shrimp.3

Foods that would purpose disorder in you or your little one (from viruses, parasites, or bacteria which include Listeria or E coli) Avoid gentle cheeses made out of unpasteurized or uncooked milk; raw cookie dough; undercooked meats, eggs, and shellfish; and deli salads. Take care in selecting and cooking lunch meats, egg dishes, and meat spreads. See greater food safety precautions throughout being pregnant External hyperlink.

Anything that isn't food some pregnant ladies may additionally want some detail that isn't food, which incorporates laundry starch, clay, ashes, or paint chips. This can also moreover constitute which you're now not receiving the proper amount of a diet. Talk for your health care practitioner if you choice something that isn't meals. He or she will be able to help you obtain the proper amount of nutrients.

Physical Activity

Should I be physical lively inside the route of my pregnancy?

Almost all ladies can and want to be physically energetic for the duration of being pregnant. According to trendy-day physical hobby suggestions External link, ordinary physical workout may also

Assist you and your toddler increase the crucial quantities of weight

Lower backaches, leg cramps, and bloating

Lower your danger for gestational diabetes (diabetes during being pregnant)

Decrease your risk for postpartum melancholy NIH outside hyperlink

There's moreover some proof that physical hobby may reduce the danger of troubles throughout pregnancy which includes preeclampsia NIH outside link (immoderate blood strain for the duration of being pregnant), reduce the period of difficult paintings and postpartum restoration, and reduce the hazard of getting a cesarean phase (or C-segment) External link.

If you had been bodily lively in advance than you have got been pregnant, you could no longer need to modify your exercise behavior. Talk together together with your fitness care professional about a manner to modify your bodily activities at some point of pregnancy.

Being physically energetic might be tough in case you don't have daycare on your different kids, haven't exercised formerly, or don't realise what to do. Keep analyzing for insights approximately how you can paintings past those problems and be bodily energetic.

Pregnant woman taking aspect in a stroll collectively with her companion and little kids.

Almost all ladies can and want to be physical energetic at some stage in being pregnant.

How plenty and what shape of bodily exercise does I need?

According to to trendy-day hints External hyperlink (PDF, 14.Four MB) , maximum ladies require the equal diploma of physical exercise that they did earlier than turning into pregnant. Aim for at the least one hundred fifty mins every week of mild-intensity cardio exercising. Aerobic sports—additionally called persistence or cardio sports activities—use massive muscular companies (again, chest, and legs) to elevate your coronary heart price and respiratory. Brisk walking is a shape of aerobic exercise.

How do you apprehend whether you're performing moderate-depth aerobic hobby? Take the "communicate test" to discover. If you're respiratory difficult but can although conduct a conversation effortlessly—however you couldn't sing—that's intermediate intensity.

If you can only utter a few terms earlier than halting for a breath, that's termed lively-depth exercise. If you were within the dependency of mission active-depth aerobic exercising or have been bodily energetic in advance than your being pregnant, then it's normally secure in case you want to preserve these sports sports at some stage in your pregnancy.

You also can chat on your health care expert approximately whether or not or no longer to or the way to alter your physical hobby at the same time as you're pregnant. If you've got were given health conditions collectively with weight issues, immoderate blood pressure, diabetes, or anemia (too few wholesome pink blood cells), touch your health care practitioner approximately a diploma of exercise that's regular for you and your unborn toddler.

How can I hold lively while pregnant?

Even if you haven't been energetic earlier than, you may be active sooner or later of your pregnancy Here are a few suggestions.

Go for a walk in which you live, at a community park, or in a retail middle with a family member or friend. If you've got already were given kids, take them with you and make it a circle of relatives adventure.

Get up and walk about at least as speedy as an hour if you take a seat down maximum of the day. When watching TV or sitting at your computer, get up and stroll approximately. Even a easy movement like taking walks in location may additionally help.

Make a technique to live lively whilst pregnant. List the belongings you'd need to adopt, which include taking walks or becoming a member of prenatal yoga magnificence. Think of the times and instances you could undertake every interest to your list, which embody first factor within the morning, all through your lunch spoil from paintings, after supper, or on Saturday afternoon. Look at your calendar or cellular phone or one-of-a-kind machine to determine the instances and times that artwork satisfactory and determine to those plans.

How can I hold secure at the identical time as being lively?

For your fitness and protection, and for your little ones, you need to now not have interaction sure strenuous sports activities at the same time as pregnant. Some of those are mentioned underneath. Talk on your health care expert about extra bodily sports activities you need to now not adopt.

Pregnant lady executes yoga stance on a yoga mat.

Prenatal yoga may be a part of your exercising plan and may lessen backaches.

Safety do's and don'ts

Follow the ones safety pointers while being lively.

Do... Don't...

Choose moderate bodily games that aren't possibly to injure you, together with strolling or water or chair aerobics. Don't take part in sports activities wherein you can fall or harm your stomach, which encompass soccer or basketball.

Drink fluids in advance than, at some point of, and after being bodily energetic. Don't overdo it. Avoid lively exercising outdoor for the duration of excessively heat climate.

Wear cushty clothing that fits well and helps and protects your breasts. Don't utilize steam rooms, warm tubs, and saunas.

Stop exercising if you feel dizzy, short of breath, exhausted, or sick in your stomach. Avoid workout routines that call for so that you can lay flat in your decrease back after week 12 for your being pregnant.

After the Baby Is Born

How can I keep healthful as soon as my teenager is born?

After you birth your toddler, your fitness can be superior if you attempt to move again to a healthy weight slowly. Not losing your "baby weight" might also additionally result in overweight or obesity later in existence. Slowly returning to a wholesome weight may additionally furthermore reduce your dangers of diabetes, coronary heart disease, and different weight-related troubles.

Healthy weight loss plan, normal bodily exercise, appropriate sleep, and special wholesome behaviors after your toddler is born may additionally assist you get higher to a healthful weight and provide you power.

After your teen is born

Consume food and liquids to in shape your calorie desires.

Regular physical exercising will keep helping your typical fitness. Moderate-depth physical workout will growth your health and can enhance your mood.

Also, physical exercising does now not appear to have bad impacts on how a brilliant deal breast milk is made, what the breast milk consists of, or how heaps the kid grows.

How also can nursing help?

Breastfeeding External hyperlink can also or won't make it less hard on the manner to shed kilos considering your frame consumes greater strength to create milk. Even if nursing does no longer help you shed pounds, it's related to numerous one-of-a-kind advantages for mother and infant.

For moms who breastfeed, medical doctors suggest External link giving their newborns completely breast milk for the number one 6 months—no different food or beverages throughout this era. Experts advocate that such mothers maintain nursing as a minimum till their infant reaches 12 months.

Calorie needs on the equal time as you're nursing rely on how an entire lot frame fats you have got had been given and how active you are. Talk along with your fitness care doctor about your calorie necessities on the same time as you are nursing.

Benefits of nursing Breastfeeding your toddler Possibly assets him or her a right balance of vitamins, minerals, and incredible crucial factors in a liquid (breast milk) that is easy to digest

Allows enhance his or her immune tool

Enables save you your youngster in opposition to commonplace ailments, such ear infections NIH outside link and diarrhea

A younger female feeds her child at her breast.

Breastfeeding gives numerous fitness benefits for mom and little one.

What else might also additionally furthermore help?

Pregnancy and the length once you transport your infant can be comfortable, exciting, emotional, disturbing, and tiring—all at once. These sensations might also additionally lead you to overeat, not collect enough power, or lose your force and power. Being type to yourself may also help you address your emotions and take a look at wholesome living practices.

Here are a few pointers that may help.

Sleep at the identical time due to the fact the little one sleeps.

Ask someone you bear in thoughts to preserve your youngster at the same time as you snooze, bathe, look at, pass for a stroll, or flow into grocery buying.

Explore organizations that you and your little one may also additionally moreover is a part of, at the facet of "new mothers" businesses.

Don't experience such as you need to accomplish all of it to your personal. Seek useful resource from pals, own family individuals, or close by help agencies.

Summary of Tips for Pregnancy

Talk in your fitness care scientific doctor approximately how a great deal weight you should advantage at some point of your being pregnant, and periodically check your development.

Consume meals and beverages excessive in folate, iron, calcium, and protein. Talk collectively with your health care expert about prenatal dietary supplements (vitamins you could take on the same time as pregnant).

Eat breakfast each day.

Eat food rich in fiber, and drink fluids (particularly water) to prevent constipation.

Avoid alcohol, uncooked or undercooked fish, fish wealthy in mercury, undercooked meat and chicken and smooth cheeses.

Do moderate-depth aerobic workout at least a hundred and fifty minutes each week in the path of your pregnancy. If you have got were given fitness troubles, talk in your health care professional earlier than you begin.

After being pregnant, often bypass again on your ordinary of common, mild-intensity bodily workout.

Gradually flow decrease lower back to a wholesome weight.

Chapter 4: Labour and Delivery

Crafting a Birth Plan

What is a starting plan?

A begin plan is a technique for you to inform your healthcare group what form of difficult paintings you'd want, what you need to expose up and what you want to keep away from. Your beginning plan might also moreover address everything concerning exertions and begin that is essential to you.

Your technique is specific to you. It will rely upon what you preference, your scientific statistics, your activities and what's to be had at your maternity service.

You don't need to write your shipping plan on a separate form, even though a few hospitals might also additionally moreover provide one you may use. You also can certainly use a piece of paper or NHS Choices provide a critical beginning plan that you could down load and fill in.

Ought I to create a shipping plan?

You do now not want to create a beginning plan. If you do determine to compose one, your midwife will can help you. They may be able to: answer your questions about what takes location in labour tell you more about what centers are available for your vicinity assist you determine out what your possibilities and priorities are.

What ought to I include in my starting plan?

You may choice to feature stuff which incorporates:

Who you need as your start companion in which you need to offer shipping

What positions you'd like to make use of for the duration of labour what type of pain comfort you need to apply within the route of labour in case you would like any music gambling even as you supply begin how you may need to supply the placenta

How you will need to feed your infant after start if you'd like several special offerings, along with a birthing pool what your alternatives are regarding spending pores and pores and skin-to-pores and pores and skin time together with your infant and no longer on time cord clamping

If you have any unique desires, together with having a signal language interpreter or you may need advantageous non secular rituals to be venerated.

After you've organized your start plan, it's a first rate idea to speak approximately it in conjunction with your begin accomplice. They is probably capable to help you better in the event that they realize greater about what you choice. It moreover allows to go about it alongside side your midwife.

If you're having a cesarean phase

There are positive topics you can upload for your start plan in case you're having a scheduled c-section. For example, you could need the screen decreased, or you couldn't need a show in any respect, so you can witness your little one being delivered. Find out greater approximately getting organized for a cesarean phase.

Vitamin K for neonates

After your infant is born, you'll be given an injection of nutrients K for them. This is indicated to assist keep away from an superb bleeding contamination referred to as Vitamin K Deficiency Bleeding.

Your midwife will chat to you approximately this injection at some stage in your pregnancy. If you don't want your little one to acquire an injection, they will take vitamins K thru mouth alternatively, but they'll require greater doses. Your midwife can also moreover provide you similarly records and you may include your choice in your transport plan.

Delayed chord clamping

NICE recommendation suggests that the umbilical twine, which attaches your placenta to the toddler, be now not clamped and severed till as a minimum 1–five mins at the same time as you supply beginning. This allows the blood from the placenta to keep being brought to the kid extended after they will be born, which assists with their increase and improvement.

Delayed cord clamping must be finished everywhere, but you should despite the fact that encompass this on your begin plan.

What takes area when I create my beginning plan?

Being flexible

Sometimes matters don't flow into in accordance to devise during pregnancy or starting. You need to be adaptable and be prepared to do matters otherwise from what you predicted. For example, a few facilities may not be handy on the day or there can be issues.

You may also moreover chat to your midwife about what would possibly take vicinity in difficult work and include your options on your start plan, but don't worry too much about searching for to encompass the whole lot. Your maternity employer wants to engage you (or your start associate if required) in any alternatives that want to be taken on the day to make certain your toddler is born nicely.

Changing your questioning

You might also additionally alternate your thoughts approximately your desires for hard work and shipping at any second, alongside sooner or later of labour in case you want to. For instance, you may apprehend on the day which you do no longer need a water beginning or which you do want fuel and air notwithstanding the whole thing.

The Wellbeing Plan

Our online health Plan is kind of a begin plan however for emotional health. It would probably assist you start thinking about the way you revel in and what assistance you could need inside the direction of your pregnancy and after the shipping.

Coping Strategies, Pain Management, and Welcoming Your Newborn

Here are eight strategies to prepare for a herbal transport enjoy.

1. Choose the suitable provider

Select a health care practitioner that is on board with herbal delivery, has experience operating with a doula, is acquainted with birthing desires, and has a low percent of cesarean deliveries. Look for a venue where experts actively engage with mother and father to ensure their delivery takes region steady with their dreams.

Nebraska Medicine nurse midwives, obstetricians, and circle of relative's treatment physicians personalize treatment to dad and mom' goals and picks We invite family human beings and doulas that will help you all through hard paintings.

If you're compelled who to chose in your shipping, that's o.K.. Watch this webinar:

Should I pick out out a medical medical doctor or a midwife?

2. Exercise regularly

You will decorate your opportunities of natural beginning with the aid of being bodily healthy. You have to exercising continuously with half of-hour of physical interest 5 to 6 days in keeping with week. Flexibility will gain you even as it comes time to push. Aim for 1/2 of-hour of prenatal yoga one or days each week.

3. Take a herbal begin class

Women who take childbirth education are much more likely to have vaginal shipping. Natural transport workshops consisting of Bradley and hypnobirthing provide strategies to address difficult artwork ache. They moreover offer you sincere expectations and encourage self notion.

Our childbirth education seminars will let you recognize what to anticipate at some point of the shipping system, especially if you're making plans a herbal beginning.

4. Hire a doula

A doula gives you assistance, encouragement, and luxury at some point of exertions and turning in. While they don't supply clinical remedy, doulas also characteristic as an endorse for you. According to a 2017 Cochrane evaluation, mothers who had non-stop tough paintings manual from a associate, midwife, or doula have been much more likely to give delivery vaginally, an entire lot less likely to require forceps or a cesarean phase, had quicker labors, and had been greater happy with their deliveries.

5. Write a start plan

A start plan is a record that specifies your hard paintings and shipping options. Women who pass into hard work with a start plan are 10% more likely to have a vaginal transport. Discuss your delivery plan together with your fitness care clinical health practitioner early to make certain that your alternatives may be fulfilled via way of your health care organization.

Nebraska Medicine physicians have one of the lowest C-segment prices in Omaha.

Make a start plan custom designed to your requirements

We can help you set up a starting plan that addresses all your necessities. Call 800.922.0000 to e-book an appointment with without a doubt virtually certainly one of our nurse midwives or obstetricians.

6. Spend early hard work at domestic

If you desire an unmediated herbal transport and a reduced C-section charge, take a look at staying power and stay home for the early a part of tough work. Most low-danger moms are stable spending early difficult earn a living from home. Keep yourself comfortable, hydrated, rested and fed. Plan on hard work being a marathon, now not a sprint. Active tough paintings begin at the same time as the cervix is dilated to form of 6 centimeters. Call your employer to determine while to are to be had.

7. Learn to confront contractions

One of the keys to an unmediated transport is being capable of loosen up in reaction to pain. Fear generates anxiety which enhances pain. If you can keep quite calm inside the midst of excessive contractions, you may have a bargain a good deal less resistance to taking off up for the child to come out. Rhythmic breathing, meditation self-hypnosis, and special rest strategies are beneficial aids for all ranges of difficult work.

8. Take use of ache manipulate techniques

There are severa of strategies that permit you to manipulate ache without using pills. Consider using any or all of those:

Chapter 5: Postpartum Journey

Natural Womanhood Logo

Many human beings find out ourselves eager to "get our bodies back" after handing over a infant. But speeding into difficult interest postpartum may additionally have immoderate repercussions, from injuries, to hormone troubles, to incontinence and more.

In the number one financial wreck of our collection on the "fourth trimester," we examined the entirety you want to understand about postpartum vitamins. Now, we're addressing the bodily issue of the early postpartum duration, concentrating on your body's actual want for rest and restoration after beginning–whether or not or not or not you introduced vaginally or with the useful resource of Cesarean phase. We furthermore cowl contemporary issues approximately postpartum exercising–while are you able to start? What types of sports are first-class at the start? What are indicators and signs which you want to touch a pelvic floor-professional physical therapist, each earlier than you restart strolling out postpartum or at the same time as you've started?

Your postpartum body desires to heal—and that entails rest

While many girls sense pressure to "bounce back" fast after their infants are born (and whether or not or no longer that stress is inner or external, perceived or genuine), in truth, women require a top notch time of relaxation. This is especially proper within the first six weeks after. Certainly, relaxing is extra tough for others. Many women should pass decrease again to paintings only a few weeks after their youngsters are born for financial or pastime protection concerns, others don't have assist annoying for their older youngsters or with home duties, and lots of others. But each female's frame wishes relaxation after her baby is delivered, and a few rest is usually better than none.

Why is relaxation so critical? For starters, hard work and shipping are physical taxing techniques, whether or now not you deliver vaginally or with the aid of the use of Cesarean segment. Your frame needs time to lighten up after what many liken to on foot a marathon. Also, as you can already recognize, irrespective of whatever manner your teen was delivered, the wound left behind through the placenta's dissociation from your endometrial can be as much as the size of a dinner plate! Along with repairing that area, you could want to get better from sutures to restore an episiotomy or a spontaneous tear skilled after a vaginal transport. Moms who undergo a C-section must heal from a number one belly operation. All of these wounds and accidents need time and rest to heal. One manner your body advises you to sluggish down or takes subjects easy is in case your lochia grows all another time (i.E. Your bleeding turns into heavier) after tapering down after your toddler's transport.

In her e-book In the Flo, hormone expert Alisa Vitti offers further incentive to take it smooth within the preliminary months postpartum.

She notes, "If you don't pay attention on your frame and try and lose the infant weight through taking region a few low-calorie weight-reduction plan and heading proper away further camp, your frame will combat once more with the resource of going into fat garage mode. Pushing yourself too hard furthermore depletes your additives of vitamins, energy, and hormones and may result in adrenal exhaustion and thyroid problems that can persist for years" (Vitti, 148).

Labor and shipping wounds or accidents apart, your muscle tissue, that have improved to two-three instances their traditional period at a few degree in the past nine+ months of your being pregnant, at the side of your ligaments, will simply require months and while masses as a year to get better. Given this, "infant frame boot camps" or one of a kind strenuous hobby completed in an try and "get your body again" inside the first few months postpartum can also additionally furthermore truly delay your healing, and run the danger of triggering incontinence (leakage of urine or stool) or pelvic organ prolapse.

Physical relaxation does embody sound asleep as a super deal as you can, but it additionally method sitting down while possible, setting your feet up, and taking pauses in among domestic sports. When you do experience the choice to get up and exercise, bypass for a piece walk. Walks are especially beneficial for girls who are enhancing from a C-segment for you to lower the risk of blood clots. You may additionally moreover strive a toddler-carrying stroll depending at the weather, or you would likely want to stroll on my own to offer yourself some alone time. Besides slight breathing and pelvic floor wearing activities, on foot is the simplest "workout" you need to be engaged in in the course of the number one six weeks, or until you've had your postpartum observe-up.

The bottom line to the diploma that you may, given your help gadget and distinct variables, relaxation as a whole lot as possible how can you tell in case you want pelvic floor physical remedy?

Every postpartum female desires to properly retrain her belly muscular tissues and rebuild her pelvic ground. You also can get securely started out out in the preliminary weeks postpartum in the consolation of your living room with those vital exercise workouts.

But at the same time as want to you're looking for expert help strengthening your pelvic floor? Lily Nichols, writer of Real Food for Pregnancy, explains alarming signs and signs for pelvic organ prolapse, which happens at the same time as your uterus, intestines, or bladder protrude down into or maybe out of the vagina. Signs that call for a expert workup embody "pressure, dragging, or fullness within the pelvic area, sensations of bulging, or the sensation of 'sitting on a ball'" (Nichols, 244). Painful sex and constipation can also be signs of a faulty pelvic floor–every of which can be addressed with the resource of pelvic ground remedy.

While any female experiencing the above signs and symptoms want to are searching out right away expert assist, Nichols honestly recommends that each one newly postpartum women are seeking advice from a girls's health physical therapist, additionally referred to as a pelvic floor therapist, in advance than resuming workout after being cleared by way in their physician, midwife, and masses of others., considering that a pelvic ground evaluation is sadly no longer a element of the 6 week visit. Pelvic ground physical therapist April Ritz concurred with Nichols, affirming Natural Womanhood:

"I distinctly endorse all postpartum moms attend as a minimum one, if no longer or 3 durations with a therapist to deal with a) the middle muscle groups (diaphragm, abdominals, pelvic floor and multifidus) b) scar mobility if a C-phase incision or perineal tearing is present c) specific posture d) lifting techniques to brace center and pelvic ground, and e) education about because it ought to be returning to exercise."

At a minimum, Ritz believes "Women with a third or fourth diploma tear need to automatically be referred for rehab postpartum" and delivered "If you are suffering with urinary incontinence after 6 weeks, tailbone ache or pelvic pain, discover a therapist near you!" If all of that isn't sufficient to inspire you to are seeking out out postpartum pelvic ground remedy, consider this: Pelvic floor bodily remedy is general-of-take care of all postpartum women in France, that is (as this text locations it) "Why French girls don't pee their pants after they laugh and also you do."

When you're prepared to start on foot out over again postpartum

If you're inquisitive about following a deliberate postpartum fitness normal, be selective! I like this one because of the truth the reason isn't weight reduction or "getting your pre-toddler frame decrease returned," but as an alternative lightly retraining your stomach muscular tissues to decorate diastasis recti (the stomach muscle separation that takes region within the majority of pregnant women) and your pelvic ground after nine-ish months of pregnancy and, for masses girls, the vaginal begin device. A rule of thumb for the number one few months postpartum is to decide on low-impact sports activities like swimming, pilates, or biking over high-impact or strenuous sports activities like something requiring jumping, kickboxing, running, and so forth. Ritz trains her sufferers that "a circulate lower again to on foot shouldn't be till 3 months postpartum at the earliest, and terrific if there may be no leakage, pelvic heaviness, or pain."

Additionally, keep away from sporting events which could get worse diastasis recti which encompass push u.S.A. Of americaor planks. When I'm in my view geared up to step by step ratchet up the exercise intensity and are looking for weight loss, I'll be looking into this

12 week plan, devised with the useful resource of a non-public teacher whose prenatal films I watched at the same time as pregnant. More beneficial material on C-phase related workout workouts can be determined right here.

So some distance, we've studied endorsed practices for maximizing vitamins and physical relaxation and restoration for the duration of the postpartum section. In our very last session, we'll look at every different pillar of postpartum nicely-being: fostering emotional fitness.

Natural Womanhood Logo

Many of us find out ourselves keen to "get our our bodies decrease returned" after delivering a child. But rushing into tough interest postpartum can also have immoderate repercussions, from accidents, to hormone issues, to incontinence and further.

In the primary economic catastrophe of our series on the "fourth trimester," we tested the entirety you need to realize approximately postpartum vitamins. Now, we're addressing the physical issue of the early postpartum length, concentrating on your body's actual want for relaxation and restoration after beginning–whether or not or now not you introduced vaginally or with the resource of Cesarean section. We also cowl popular issues approximately postpartum exercising–while are you able to begin? What forms of sports activities are fine on the begin? What are caution signs and symptoms and signs and symptoms that you ought to contact a pelvic ground-knowledgeable physical therapist, every earlier than you restart operating out postpartum or while you've commenced?

Your postpartum frame needs to heal–and that includes rest

While many ladies feel strain to "bounce back" speedy after their toddlers are born (and whether or not that strain is internal or outside, perceived or authentic), in fact, ladies require a huge time of relaxation. This is mainly real in the first six weeks after. Certainly, exciting is greater hard for others. Many women need to cross lower back to work just a few weeks after their children are born for economic or interest safety problems, others don't have assist being involved for their older kids or with home obligations, and so on. But every female's body dreams rest after her infant is delivered, and some relaxation is continuously better than none.

Why is rest so critical? For starters, labour and shipping are bodily taxing procedures, whether or not you deliver vaginally or with the aid of way of Caesarean phase. Your frame dreams time to loosen up after what many liken to taking walks a marathon. Also, as you could already comprehend, no matter some element way your infant became brought, the wound left in the returned of via the placenta's dissociation out of your endometrium can be as much as the size of a dinner plate! Along with repairing that area, you can need to get nicely from sutures to repair an episiotomy or a spontaneous tear experienced after a vaginal starting. Moms who undergo a C-phase need to heal from a number one belly operation. All of these wounds and injuries want time and rest to heal. One manner your frame advises you to gradual down or take subjects smooth is if your lochia grows another time (i.E. Your bleeding becomes heavier) after tapering down after your infant's shipping.

In her ebook In the Flo, hormone professional Alisa Vitti gives in addition incentive to take it clean inside the preliminary months postpartum. She notes, "If you don't listen in your frame and attempt to lose the child weight via occurring some low-calorie food regimen and heading proper away in addition camp, your body will fight lower again with the useful aid of going into fat storage mode. Pushing yourself too hard additionally depletes your additives of vitamins, power, and hormones and might motive adrenal exhaustion and thyroid troubles which could persist for years" (Vitti, 148).

Labor and shipping wounds or accidents aside, your muscular tissues, that have prolonged to two-3 instances their well-known duration sooner or later of the beyond nine+ months of your pregnancy, collectively at the side of your ligaments, will absolutely require months or whilst a amazing deal as a one year to recover. Given this, "little one frame boot camps" or wonderful strenuous interest completed in a try to "get your body back" inside the first few months postpartum may additionally truly take away your restoration, and run the chance of triggering incontinence (leakage of urine or stool) or pelvic organ prolapse.

Physical relaxation does include napping as loads as you could, but it moreover technique sitting down while possible, putting your ft up, and taking pauses in amongst home activities. When you do sense the choice to rise up and workout, move for a hint walk.

Walks are in particular useful for ladies who're improving from a C-section as a way to lower the threat of blood clots. You may additionally furthermore attempt a toddler-sporting walk relying on the weather, or you may possibly need to walk on my own to provide yourself some on my own time. Besides slight respiratory and pelvic floor wearing occasions, taking walks is the handiest "exercising" you need to be engaged in subsequently of the number one six weeks, or until you've had your postpartum observe-up.

The backside line to the degree that you may, given your help tool and distinctive variables, rest as an lousy lot as possible.

How are you able to tell in case you want pelvic floor bodily remedy?

Every postpartum female desires to well retrain her belly muscle companies and rebuild her pelvic ground. You may also moreover get securely started out in the preliminary weeks postpartum within the consolation of your living room with those simple workout physical activities.

But at the same time as ought to you're looking for expert assist strengthening your pelvic ground? Lily Nichols, author of Real Food for Pregnancy, explains alarming signs and signs for pelvic organ prolapse, which takes place while your uterus, intestines, or bladder protrude down into or perhaps out of the vagina. Signs that call for a expert workup include "pressure, dragging, or fullness within the pelvic vicinity, sensations of bulging, or the sensation of 'sitting on a ball'" (Nichols, 244). Painful sex and constipation can also be symptoms of a defective pelvic ground—every of which can be addressed via pelvic floor treatment.

While any woman experiencing the above symptoms have to are attempting to find for right away expert assist, Nichols in truth recommends that all newly postpartum ladies are seeking out recommendation from a girls's health physical therapist, additionally known as a pelvic ground therapist, in advance than resuming workout after being cleared by using manner of the usage of their physician, midwife, and many others., thinking about that a pelvic ground evaluation is lamentably not a factor of the 6 week visit.

"I instead advise all postpartum mothers attend at the least one, if not or 3 training with a therapist to cope with a) the center muscle mass (diaphragm, abdominals, pelvic floor and multifidus) b) scar mobility if a C-section incision or perineal tearing is gift c) real posture d) lifting strategies to brace center and pelvic floor, and e) training about efficiently returning to exercise."

At a minimal, Ritz believes "Women with a third or fourth degree tear have to automatically be referred for rehab postpartum" and introduced "If you're suffering with urinary incontinence after 6 weeks, tailbone pain or pelvic pain, find a therapist near you!" If all of that isn't enough to encourage you to searching for out postpartum pelvic floor treatment, maintain in thoughts this: Pelvic floor physical remedy is stylish-of-care for all postpartum ladies in France, it actually is (as these article locations it) "Why French ladies don't pee their pants after they laugh and you do."

When you're prepared to start working out another time postpartum

If you're interested by following a planned postpartum health recurring, be selective! I like this one due to the fact the goal is not weight loss or "getting your pre-infant frame decrease again," but as an alternative lightly retraining your belly muscle groups to enhance diastasis recti (the stomach muscle separation that occurs inside the majority of pregnant girls) and your pelvic floor after 9-ish months of pregnancy and, for masses women, the vaginal begin technique. A rule of thumb for the number one few months postpartum is to pick low-impact sporting activities like swimming, pilates, or cycling over immoderate-effect or strenuous sports like a few element requiring jumping, kickboxing, jogging, and so on. Ritz trains her sufferers that "a pass again to taking walks shouldn't be till 3 months postpartum on the earliest, and most effective if there can be no leakage, pelvic heaviness, or ache."

Additionally, avoid wearing events which can get worse diastasis recti such as push u.S.Or planks. When I'm for my part prepared to grade by grade ratchet up the exercise intensity and are searching out weight loss, I'll be looking into this 12 week plan, devised by using way of a personal trainer whose prenatal videos I watched while pregnant.

Chapter 6: Preparing For a Natural Pregnancy

Assessing Your Readiness

Knowing your readiness level is crucial in growing a a success and healthful environment for each you and your infant. Before embarking on a herbal being pregnant adventure, it's far essential to recognize the importance of getting a healthful body. It's crucial to examine your cycle, fertility symptoms, and blessings of prenatal nutrients earlier than conceiving evidently. Understanding those additives will assist you create a exceptional surroundings for thought and a wholesome being pregnant.

1. Your Menstrual Cycle: A everyday menstrual cycle is the foundation of top fertility. If your intervals are abnormal or absent, it is probably tough to decide your fertile window. In such instances, are looking for steering from a healthcare professional to address functionality underlying motives.

2.   Fertility Signs: Tracking ovulation signs and symptoms like modifications in cervical mucus, basal body temperature (BBT), or ovulation ache will let you determine your fertile times. You can use those symptoms to devise for concept within the course of those maximum pleasant days.

three. Prenatal Vitamins: Start taking prenatal vitamins in advance than attempting notion. Folic acid is especially crucial in some unspecified time in the future of early pregnancy to prevent neural tube defects in growing infants. Consult your healthcare issuer for suggestions on prenatal nutrients appropriate for you.

Mental training is actually as crucial as bodily readiness. Acknowledging the following elements of intellectual coaching will let you navigate the herbal pregnancy journey with greater self perception.

1.   Stress Management: Chronic strain may additionally additionally negatively impact fertility and standard fitness. It's

crucial to control stress effectively via meditation, yoga, or rest strategies that paintings brilliant for you.

2. Support System: Building a strong assist machine of buddies, own family, and applicable professionals is critical while getting equipped for a natural being pregnant adventure. Seek advice from those who've professional herbal pregnancies, and percentage your mind and feelings brazenly.

3. Setting Realistic Expectations: Recognize that concept may not display up proper away and that each pregnancy is one-of-a-kind. It's critical to set realistic expectations and stay affected man or woman at some stage in the gadget.

four. Healthcare Provider Relationship: Establish a relationship with a healthcare corporation professional in herbal pregnancy care. This guarantees regular guidance in the path of your being pregnant journey.

Emotional readiness is crucial in developing a loving and supportive environment to your developing infant. Consider those additives of emotional preparedness:

1.   Communication: Open conversation along with your associate about expectancies, fears, and parenting philosophies is essential at the equal time as making ready for a natural pregnancy. Engaging in conversations can help every companions recognize every different's dreams and perspectives.

2.   Managing Emotions: Pregnancy can be an emotional rollercoaster, with hormonal shifts inflicting mood modifications. Understanding this reality will let you manage feelings better during pregnancy.

three. Trying Consciously: Be aware about all feelings related to looking to conceive. Acknowledge capability anxiety or apprehension related to concept tries. This awareness permits you to manipulate any horrible feelings better amidst the journey.

4.   Addressing Past Traumas: If you have got experienced beyond traumas which includes miscarriage, stillbirth, or fertility worrying conditions, it is essential to address lingering feelings in training for a current pregnancy adventure. Speak with a therapist or depended on confidant to help manipulate those complicated feelings.

Certain life-style adjustments can considerably enhance your fertility and everyday fitness throughout the herbal being pregnant adventure:

1.   Nutrition: A healthy weight loss plan rich in end result, veggies, lean proteins, entire grains, and healthy fat is important for pinnacle-awesome fertility. Avoid processed factors, immoderate caffeine, or alcohol intake even as looking for to conceive.

2.   Exercise: Regular moderate exercise lets in normal health, reduces stress levels, and prepares your body for being pregnant. Consult your healthcare enterprise

organisation on suitable exercising regimens suitable in your fitness degree.

three. Weight Management: Being underweight or overweight can negatively effect fertility. Aim for a healthful weight that falls within the regular BMI variety to decorate your possibilities of conceiving.

Partner Involvement and Support

In a natural being pregnant guide, it's miles vital to emphasise that each companions want to be actively involved in choice-making concerning prenatal care, tough paintings, and delivery. This involvement can manual the bond among the couple and create a enjoy of concord and shared duty for the trendy lifestyles they may be bringing into the arena. Providing emotional help, sharing records, accompanying every one-of-a-type to prenatal appointments, and discussing begin alternatives collectively can help set the degree for a healthful herbal pregnancy revel in.

1. Emotional Support: Providing emotional useful resource at some stage in pregnancy is crucial in ensuring a pleasant and nurturing environment for each companions. Emotional adjustments are commonplace in some unspecified time in the future of pregnancy due to fluctuating hormone tiers. These fluctuations can bring about mood swings, anxiety, despair, or emotions of self-doubt for some pregnant people. A supportive associate who listens empathetically, offers reassurance, and helps preserve optimism can help deplete those horrible feelings.

Partners can inspire self-care with the useful resource of sharing normal relaxation sports activities together with meditation or gentle sporting sports activities like prenatal yoga or on foot collectively. Creating a safe location for open conversation about fears, expectations, and destiny plans will supply a boost to the partnership in the path of this adventure.

2. Sharing Information: Both partners want to be prepared and informed about the severa factors of natural pregnancy to make nicely-informed alternatives together. Researching topics together with nutrients, dietary nutritional dietary supplements, shipping strategies, midwives, doulas, childbirth education training in advance than making joint alternatives will make contributions to a shared expertise of your desired technique at some point of this specific revel in.

Staying updated with the modern statistics in prenatal care – such as staying informed on herbal pain consolation strategies, final fetal positioning, and pregnancy-regular remedies – will help every companions navigate the herbal pregnancy adventure with self notion and competence.

three. Accompanying Each Other to Prenatal Appointments: Prenatal appointments are essential for monitoring the health and development of every the expectant mom and her developing baby. Partner involvement in prenatal visits reinforces help via offering a deeper know-how of the being pregnant approach, improving communication, and familiarity with the healthcare crew.

By attending appointments collectively, companions can live engaged inside the pregnancy manner, ask questions, percentage issues, and display their determination to the shared experience. Partners emerge as more knowledgeable, which enhances their capability to provide informed support as they expect their new roles as parents.

4. Discussing Birth Preferences: As you technique your start date, it's essential to talk about your alternatives collectively together with your associate in detail. This talk should remember topics related to labor induction, pain consolation options, childbirth positions, breastfeeding selections, postpartum care, and plenty of greater. Together you could draft a starting plan that caters for your dreams for a natural enjoy.

Ensure that your partner is also privy to your chosen coping mechanisms sooner or later of hard paintings and whilst high-quality interventions can be suitable. By having those conversations in advance of time, your companion can better advise on your desires in the route of hard work.

five. Preparing for New Parenthood Roles: Embracing parenthood is a existence-converting revel in that includes its proportion of stressful situations and rewards. To better put together themselves for their roles as dad and mom and partners-in-parenting, couples must engage in open verbal exchange about their man or woman expectations from every unique in advance than the kid arrives.

In addition to attending childbirth training schooling together or taking parenting guides on line or in-individual, discussing duties department including feeding schedules (if breastfeeding or bottle-feeding), diapering responsibilities, nighttime wakings – will help set expectancies for every companion's involvement in traumatic for the kid.

Finding the Right Healthcare Provider

With such a whole lot of alternatives to be had, it could be overwhelming to find the high-quality healthy to your private opportunities and goals. This phase will guide you thru the manner of locating the healthcare enterprise that suits you brilliant, making sure that your pregnancy experience is as easy and interesting as feasible.

1. Identifying Your Priorities: Before embarking on your look for the right healthcare company, take the time to keep in mind and prioritize your personal values and desires. Write down what subjects most to you and speak together with your companion or help system. Some common picks encompass:

Natural childbirth manual

Accessibility of care

Reputation and revel in

Affordability and insurance insurance

Personal connection and communique

Keeping those priorities in thoughts will assist you're making greater knowledgeable alternatives at some stage in your search for a healthcare issuer that enables your herbal pregnancy goals.

2. Researching Different Types of Providers: There are severa kinds of healthcare providers that specialize in pregnancy and childbirth, each with their particular strategies to care. Understanding these variations will let you choose a expert who aligns collectively together with your personal ideals and dreams for a herbal being pregnant. Some commonplace options embody:

a) Obstetricians: Medical clinical doctors who specialise in pregnancy, hard art work, and transport, OBs usually paintings internal hospital settings. They may not attention as an entire lot on natural pregnancies however can manipulate excessive-hazard pregnancies and complicated deliveries.

b) Certified Nurse-Midwives: Registered nurses with superior schooling in midwifery frequently emphasize natural starting practices at the same time as providing ordinary prenatal, labor, shipping, and postpartum care in each medical institution settings or birth centers.

c) Direct-Entry Midwives: Non-nurse midwives who whole midwifery training through apprenticeships or self-check can be specially focused on herbal starting in low-hazard pregnancies. They normally attend births at houses or start centers.

Research the varieties of providers available in your place and go through in thoughts attending pregnancy assist corporations or training to acquire private reviews and recommendations from wonderful expectant moms.

three. Asking the Right Questions: Once you've got were given narrowed down your options, time table consultations with capacity vendors to determine if their method aligns collectively with your options. Prepare a list of questions to cover at a few level inside the ones conversations, along with:

a) What is your philosophy regarding herbal childbirth expectancies and control of potential complications?

b) How do you aid comfort measures inside the direction of hard art work, which includes water remedy, massage, or meditation practices?

c) Do you inspire tough work training and doula guide?

d) What are your hints on ordinary prenatal screening and attempting out?

e) In case of critical clinical interventions, what options do you endorse for a more natural enjoy?

116

Remember that the tremendous healthcare organization for you is someone who shares your values and is open to discussing your wishes for a natural pregnancy journey.

four. Considering Accessibility and Environment: Aspects collectively with sanatorium vicinity, hours, coverage compatibility, and birthing facility alternatives are critical to keep in thoughts while deciding on a healthcare corporation. Ensure that their workplace is pretty simply located and that they accept your insurance plan.

Additionally, find out the facilities wherein you need to provide beginning. Hospital settings ought to probably provide extra era and belongings in case of complications but can be a great deal less conducive to a herbal birthing revel in because of strict protocols. Birth facilities or domestic births often offer a greater comfortable surroundings centered on empowering herbal childbirth however may lack instant access to complete hospital therapy if emergencies stand up.

5. Listening to Your Intuition: Finally, believe your intestine instinct at the identical time as deciding on a healthcare issuer. After accumulating information and meeting with functionality applicants, mirror on the interactions, and decide which one feels just like the first-rate in shape for you. Feeling supported and consistent for your choice will make contributions certainly to your common pregnancy journey.

Chapter 7: Navigating the First Trimester

Coping with Morning Sickness and Fatigue

Morning sickness and fatigue are commonplace signs women experience at some stage in the primary trimester of pregnancy. Although those symptoms can be tough, there are various natural techniques to help decrease their impact to your life. Below are severa procedures to address morning illness and fatigue at a few degree inside the number one trimester.

1. Nutrition: One of the crucial additives of coping with morning contamination is being aware about your nutrition. Pregnancy will growth your frame's call for for nutrients, so it is vital to consume a healthy, balanced food plan with lots of culmination, veggies, whole grains, and lean proteins. Eating smaller meals at some stage in the day can assist prevent surprising bouts of nausea. Also, taking a prenatal nutrients with folic acid may moreover moreover beautify your commonplace well-being finally of this period.

2. Hydration: Staying well-hydrated is important to your wellknown fitness and can also assist alleviate morning illness. Sipping water at some stage inside the day guarantees that you're converting fluids out of place due to vomiting or perspiration. You can pick out extraordinary hydrating liquids like herbal tea or broths if simple water seems unappealing.

three. Ginger: Ginger has been used by pregnant women round the world for loads of years to soothe nausea related to morning infection. You can upload smooth ginger on your food or try ginger dietary supplements, snacks, or tea to securely encompass it into your every day ordinary.

4. Acupressure: Applying pressure to the P6 acupoint—located on the inner wrist—can assist alleviate nausea and vomiting related to morning infection. You can gently press this factor your self or buy a wristband particularly designed for nausea comfort.

five. Aromatherapy: Inhaling advantageous essential oils like peppermint, lemon, or lavender oil can also assist lessen emotions of nausea and encourage rest for the duration of moments of fatigue. Remember pleasant to apply great oils and keep away from applying them right away onto your pores and pores and skin.

6. Rest: Fatigue is a herbal a part of pregnancy, in particular inside the first trimester as your body undergoes huge modifications. Listening in your body and taking the time to relaxation is critical. Don't revel in accountable if you need a snooze or extra sleep—your frame calls for it to maintain your health and the properly-being of your little one.

7. Gentle Exercise: While rest is vital, challenge slight exercising like prenatal yoga, walking, or swimming can assist alleviate fatigue and boom your power tiers. Exercise moreover promotes wholesome movement,

that could assist with nausea and mood swings.

eight. Create a Supportive Environment: Your surroundings can substantially effect your pressure levels, which could exacerbate morning infection and fatigue signs and signs and symptoms. Make an attempt to create a calming environment at domestic via the use of decluttering, incorporating soothing scents, and ensuring you have got comfortable spots to loosen up.

9. Adjust Your Schedule: If you discover that morning infection or fatigue are mainly disruptive at positive times of the day, keep in thoughts adjusting your each day time table as a end result. For instance, you could want to deal with vital responsibilities while you're feeling most lively or take breaks within the direction of intervals of drowsiness.

10. Emotional Support: Connecting with others who recognize what you're going via— whether or not or no longer or not it's far circle of relatives, friends, or online help

agencies—can provide treasured emotional guide in the course of this difficult time. Don't hesitate to are looking for for professional assist from a being pregnant counselor if wanted for coping with the emotional components of these signs and symptoms and signs.

eleven. Seeking Medical Attention: In some times, morning sickness and fatigue may also moreover moreover end up severe and require scientific intervention. Don't hesitate to talk about in conjunction with your healthcare provider if you're experiencing prolonged bouts of vomiting or in case your signs and symptoms and signs seem insufferable.

Nutrition and Dietary Choices

Nourishing your frame with healthful food choices is critical to assist the increase and improvement of your infant. During the number one trimester, your nutritional goals will shift, and it is critical to understand what to eat for high-quality dietary assist. Let's find out nutritious components, dietary adjustments, and tips for handling common first-trimester traumatic conditions.

1. Nutrient-Dense Foods: In the first trimester, it's miles extra important than ever to devour nutrient-dense meals that provide the critical vitamins and minerals your child wants to broaden nicely. Some of these key nutrients embody folic acid, iron, calcium, nutrients D, and protein. Here are a few examples of nutrient-dense substances:

a) Leafy Greens: Spinach and kale are brilliant property of folic acid, iron, and calcium.

b) Fish: Choose low-mercury fish like salmon or sardines for a lift of omega-3 fatty acids critical for mind development.

c) Eggs: A bendy protein-packed opportunity that incorporates essential nutrients like choline.

d) Legumes: Beans, chickpeas, and lentils are brilliant belongings of iron and protein.

e) Nuts and Seeds: Almonds and chia seeds are a awesome way to add calcium, healthful fats, and fiber.

f) Yogurt: Choose simple Greek yogurt for an notable deliver of calcium and protein.

2. The Importance of Prenatal Vitamins: While a balanced weight-reduction plan is normally best in the route of pregnancy, prenatal vitamins can assist fill in the gaps to ensure you are getting enough vital vitamins. Look for a prenatal vitamins containing folic acid to prevent begin defects, iron to help stepped forward blood amount in pregnancy, and nutrients D for immune help. Take them as prescribed with the resource of your healthcare issuer.

three. Managing Morning Sickness: Many ladies enjoy morning contamination throughout the primary trimester. As a end result, it may be hard to stick to a nutritious food plan. Try those guidelines to help control your symptoms and signs and symptoms:

a) Keep crackers or dry cereal with the aid of your mattress and eat a small amount earlier than getting up in the morning.

b) Eat smaller, more frequent meals at some stage in the day.

c) Sip ginger tea or ginger ale made with actual ginger to assuage an disillusioned belly.

d) Stay hydrated and drink water at a few degree inside the day.

e) Avoid overly fragrant, surprisingly spiced, or greasy components that can purpose nausea.

4. Dietary Changes: You also can word changes to your urge for meals or food alternatives at some stage in the number one trimester. Some girls crave specific meals, even as others also can expand aversions to previously cherished gadgets. While it's vital to nourish your body, do now not pressure an excessive amount of about those quick adjustments. It's more vital to pay attention

for your body and devour a balanced weight-reduction plan in which viable.

5. Foods to Avoid: Some substances bring extra chance at some point of pregnancy and should be avoided or confined:

a) Raw or undercooked eggs, meat, and fish

b) High-mercury fish together with swordfish, shark, and king mackerel

c) Unpasteurized milk or cheese

d) Deli meats, except heated till steaming warmness

e) Excessive caffeine (restrict intake to two hundred mg consistent with day)

6. Promoting a Healthy Lifestyle: In addition to being attentive to your diet regime in the course of the primary trimester, don't forget implementing a few healthy way of life practices:

a) Engage in slight workout like taking walks or prenatal yoga

b) Prioritize sleep and intention for as a minimum 7 hours consistent with night time time time

c) Avoid alcohol and smoking (together with secondhand smoke)

d) Practice relaxation techniques like deep respiration or meditation

e) Stay linked with friends and family for emotional assist in your adventure

Gentle Exercises for Early Pregnancy

As you navigate through the early ranges of your pregnancy, staying active and keeping a healthy lifestyle can drastically benefit both you and your growing child. In this phase, we will communicate mild bodily games which can be appropriate for women in their first trimester of being pregnant. These bodily video games can help to alleviate not unusual discomforts, improve your mood, and promote usual properly-being, making it an critical part of your natural being pregnant adventure.

However, in advance than embarking on any workout software at some point of being pregnant, it's miles important to first visit your healthcare business enterprise to make sure which you are making secure options for your self and your unborn little one.

1. Prenatal Yoga: Prenatal yoga is one of the great sorts of workout inside the path of early being pregnant. It permits to promote relaxation, flexibility, and energy at the equal time as additionally education you right breathing strategies. Many poses and stretches goal unique muscle corporations that can relieve anxiety inside the once more, hips, and pelvis – regions in which pregnant girls often enjoy pain.

If you're new to yoga or have in no manner practiced it in advance than, maintain in mind becoming a member of a prenatal yoga class as the teachers can guide you through the changed poses tailor-made for pregnant ladies.

2. Walking: Walking is a low-effect aerobic workout that calls for no precise machine and can be loved with the beneficial aid of people of all fitness tiers. This hobby encourages wholesome weight benefit and stepped forward flow into throughout pregnancy whilst moreover presenting an opportunity to live linked with nature or enjoy quality time with friends and circle of relatives.

Start with a slow and ordinary pace, step by step growing the period of your walks as desired. Pay hobby for your body's indicators and relaxation on the equal time as vital.

3. Pelvic tilt bodily video games: Pelvic tilt physical video games are incredible for strengthening your center muscle groups, so you can display invaluable while wearing the extra weight of your growing child. They furthermore useful resource in alleviating lower once more pain as they assist maintain right alignment during being pregnant.

To carry out a pelvic tilt: Lie on your again, ft flat and shoulder-width aside, collectively at the side of your knees bent. Inhale deeply and then exhale, tilting your pelvis upwards thru contracting your belly muscle tissue. Hold the vicinity for a few seconds after which release.

four. Swimming: Swimming is an awesome low-effect exercising for pregnant women because it gives a complete-frame exercise with out putting any stress to your joints. The buoyancy of the water allows your growing stomach, allowing you to transport without a trouble and splendor.

Always select a pool with warm water to save you muscle cramping or pain resulting from unexpected temperature changes. Avoid immoderate-intensity sports activities sports like diving, leaping off systems, or taking element in touch water sports sports.

5. Seated leg lifts: Seated leg lifts help to tone and decorate the muscle tissues for your thighs and buttocks on the identical time as also providing a few treatment for decrease once more pain.

To carry out a seated leg deliver: Sit on a chair with each toes flat at the ground. Keeping one foot planted on the ground for stability, slowly growth the alternative leg at once out in front of you until it's miles parallel with the ground. Hold for a few seconds in advance than decreasing it backpedal.

6. Arm curls: First-trimester arm curls are satisfactory for retaining better frame electricity and may be performed the use of mild dumbbells or perhaps stuffed water bottles.

To perform an arm curl: Hold the weights thru the use of your facets with fingers going through beforehand. Bend your elbows to carry the weights inside the path of your shoulders at the same time as maintaining your better hands desk bound. Lower them back off to the start feature.

Chapter 8: Thriving Through the Second Trimester

Embracing Your Changing Body

As you enter the second trimester of your being pregnant, you may note many speedy and huge modifications to your frame. It's a time of transformation and adjustment, and embracing the ones modifications is crucial to maintaining a super outlook in your natural pregnancy journey. Here, we are going to provide pointers on a way to include your changing body inside the direction of this segment, so that you can feel assured, healthy, and related together along with your infant.

1. Acknowledge Your Physical Changes: In the second one trimester, your toddler will grow brief, and so will your body. You will gain weight and experience an increasing stomach in addition to extended breast period. Instead of evaluating your self to others or striving for unrealistic expectancies, widely recognized and accept these modifications as signs and

133

symptoms which you're nurturing a state-of-the-art lifestyles inner of you.

2. Stay Active: Maintaining a everyday exercising recurring in the direction of the second trimester can benefit each you and your infant. Staying active at some stage in this time can help you preserve a healthful weight gain, increase electricity degrees, deliver a lift to muscles for difficult work and delivery, or perhaps alleviate a few commonplace being pregnant discomforts like backaches. Consult together together with your healthcare provider to decide stable exercising bodily sports that work first rate for you.

three. Dress for Comfort: As your frame maintains to change throughout the second one trimester, you may locate that a few devices for your material cloth cabinet no longer fit without issue or flatteringly. Invest in maternity apparel designed to residence your developing belly or bear in thoughts repurposing wonderful snug alternatives like stretchy pants and prolonged skirts.

4. Nurture Your Skin: During the second one trimester, hormonal changes also can motive the pores and pores and skin to your belly to stretch as your uterus expands to address the growing fetus. Stay properly-hydrated and moisturize frequently with natural merchandise designed for pregnant ladies to reduce itching or particular pores and skin discomforts.

five. Maintain Proper Posture: As your toddler bump grows during the second trimester, your middle of gravity will shift, which also can motive pressure to your lower once more. Be conscious of your posture, mainly on the identical time as sitting or recognition for extended durations. Consider incorporating slight stretches and energy training sports activities activities that target posture enhancement.

6. Connect with Your Baby: With each week and new being pregnant milestone, you've

got emerge as greater linked to the little life developing inner of you. Part of accepting the ones adjustments is constantly celebrating this bond on the facet of your baby. Feeling their first moves sooner or later of this trimester may be an interesting and emotional revel in that in addition connects you for your being pregnant adventure.

7. Seek Support from Loved Ones: Whether it's miles your partner, friends, or fellow expectant mothers, sharing your studies in the course of the second one trimester can offer emotional consolation as you navigate this phase. Openly speak your converting body and are trying to find guide from others who understand and empathize with what you're going thru.

8. Practice Self-Care: Prioritize self-care at some point of the second one trimester through having a healthful healthy dietweight-reduction plan, proper sleep, and strain-decreasing sports like prenatal yoga or meditation. These practices promote no

longer only physical wellness however furthermore intellectual well-being as they help you take shipping of a converting body with calmness and gratitude.

9. Capture the Memories: Embracing the changes all through your second trimester moreover technique cherishing each 2nd of this exquisite experience. Snap images or maintain a pregnancy mag to look again on and keep in mind how sturdy and extraordinary your frame turned into throughout this time.

10. Focus on the Positive: Lastly, preserve a splendid outlook inside the direction of all the adjustments within the 2d trimester via focusing on the terrific reality that your frame is nurturing a ultra-modern-day lifestyles interior it. It's essential to remind oneself that those changes are taking location for a cause – making equipped each you and your child for a wholesome existence collectively.

Staying Active and Fit

The second trimester is regularly taken into consideration the golden period of being pregnant. As you circulate this diploma, morning illness and fatigue can also moreover begin to subside, permitting you to experience a renewed feel of energy and strength. As you maintain your journey in the direction of motherhood, it's far crucial to preserve yourself physically energetic and healthful.

1. Choose Appropriate Exercises: During the second trimester, your frame undergoes numerous modifications as your infant grows. It's important to choose out low-effect bodily sports that do not impose more stress for your joints or pelvic floor muscle corporations. Some exquisite picks for staying wholesome encompass:

a) Prenatal yoga: This low-effect exercise is incredible for boosting flexibility, stability, and strength at the same time as preserving you cushty and targeted.

b) Swimming or water aerobics: Being inside the water takes the load off your developing belly, offering remedy from pressure on your joints and backbone.

c) Brisk walks: Walking is a easy and effective manner to preserve cardiovascular health on the equal time as mitigating the threat of harm.

Always communicate over with your healthcare provider in advance than starting any new exercise everyday for the duration of pregnancy.

2. Maintain Proper Posture: As your little one grows in length at some degree inside the 2d one trimester, retaining right posture will become increasingly critical. Carrying greater weight can adjust your body's center of gravity and motive stress on your decrease once more muscle tissues. When popularity or sitting, attention on maintaining your backbone aligned by using manner of the use of straightening up with shoulders pulled

back, chest open, and pelvis tilted beforehand.

three. Modify Your Exercise Routines: As your pregnancy progresses, you have to regulate positive factors of your exercise workouts. Avoid sports that placed immoderate stress for your joints or increase the threat of damage, which incorporates contact sports activities sports or excessive-intensity interval schooling (HIIT). Adapt carrying activities to fit your frame's desires through way of the use of useful resource gadgets together with pillows or workout balls for balance and luxury.

four. Strengthen Your Pelvic Floor Muscles: Pregnancy places multiplied strain at the pelvic ground muscular tissues, which useful resource your uterus, bladder, and bowels, likely resulting in incontinence and prolapse. Strengthening those muscular tissues with the beneficial useful resource of working in the direction of Kegel sporting sports activities can advantage you in the route of being pregnant and after childbirth. To perform Kegels, settlement the muscular tissues you use to prevent urine go with the flow for 3-five 2d durations, often developing to ten seconds. Aim for 10 to fifteen repetitions, 3 instances an afternoon.

5. Pay Attention to Your Body's Signals: Your frame undergoes huge adjustments in the course of being pregnant; therefore, it is essential to pay attention to what it is telling you. Pay interest to signs such as fatigue, shortness of breath, or dizziness that may propose immoderate exertion or dehydration. Take everyday breaks finally of workout training and make sure appropriate enough hydration via ingesting plenty of water.

6. Fuel Your Body with Healthy Nutrition: A wholesome diet plays a important role in preserving your electricity stages and imparting vitamins on your developing toddler. Focus on ingesting nutrient-dense foods alongside aspect fruits, veggies, lean proteins, whole grains, and wholesome fat at

the identical time as restricting processed elements and sensitive sugars.

7. Stay Motivated: Staying lively at some stage in pregnancy is essential for each your bodily and intellectual well-being; but, it can be hard to keep motivation. Set precise fitness goals which includes taking walks for half-hour every day or attending prenatal yoga schooling two instances in step with week. Celebrate your achievements and discover support from pals or family folks who can maintain you accountable.

eight. Embrace Relaxation Techniques: Incorporating rest techniques into your day by day recurring can restriction stress at the equal time as selling emotional wellness. Meditation, deep respiration carrying sports, and mindfulness practices foster a feel of inner peace and balance within the route of your being pregnant journey.

Nutritional Needs for You and Your Baby

As you input the second trimester of your pregnancy, you will be conscious that your frame has began to adapt to the changes to cope with your growing child. Along with this, your nutritional desires may additionally even growth sooner or later of this period. It's critical to keep a healthy eating regimen to guide your toddler's improvement and provide you with the energy you want for a natural being pregnant. In this segment, we are capable to speak the severa dietary desires for you and your baby via the second one trimester.

1. Macronutrients:

a) Protein: Protein is a vital nutrient in some unspecified time in the future of being pregnant, helping the boom and improvement of your little one's organs, muscle companies, and tissues. Make incredible to embody lean meat (like hen and turkey), fish (specifically salmon and top notch fatty fish), eggs, dairy merchandise (like yogurt and cheese), lentils, beans, tofu, quinoa, or nuts for your day by day meal plan. Aim for approximately 71g of protein in keeping with day in the path of this trimester.

b) Carbohydrates: Whole grains are an important deliver of strength for every you and your little one. They provide fiber, which aids digestion and facilitates with stopping gestational diabetes and constipation. Choose whole wheat bread, brown rice, quinoa, barley, oats together with fruits and veggies as wholesome belongings of carbohydrates.

c) Healthy fat: Healthy fats are critical in your toddler's brain improvement and hormonal production. Foods rich in omega-three fatty acids like walnuts, chia seeds, flaxseeds, and fish like salmon are superb assets of these healthful fat.

2. Micronutrient wishes:

a) Folate: Continue taking folic acid within the route of the entirety of your second trimester to prevent neural tube defects to your child. Good resources embody darkish leafy vegetables like spinach or kale, fortified cereals or pasta, beans or lentils.

b) Iron: As your blood extent will boom all through being pregnant, your iron necessities turn out to be extra huge. Ensure to embody iron-wealthy elements inclusive of spinach, beans, lentils, tofu, lean meats, and iron-fortified cereals for your every day consumption. Pair people with Vitamin C assets like oranges or bell peppers to beautify iron absorption.

c) Calcium: During being pregnant, calcium is specially critical for developing the infant's bones and tooth. Dairy merchandise like milk, cheese, yogurt, and leafy vegetables like kale and bok choy are tremendous calcium assets. Aim for 1,000 mg of calcium every day.

d) Vitamin D: Vitamin D works along aspect calcium to assemble and preserve healthy bones and enamel for every you and your little one. Sun publicity can provide you with food plan D; however, it's miles critical to get enough from food belongings as well. Foods like eggs, fish like salmon or sardines, cheese, or fortified milk are notable assets of Vitamin D.

3. Hydration: Staying well-hydrated is vital at some point of being pregnant as it helps maintain proper digestive health and aids in the absorption of nutrients. Aim for eight to ten glasses of water every day at the facet of various hydrating fluids which incorporates natural teas or coconut water.

four. Breakfast thoughts: Kick-off your day with a nutritious breakfast that consists of a balance of carbohydrates, proteins, and fat on the factor of give up result or vegetables. Some examples embody avocado toast with eggs or smoked salmon on complete-grain bread; Greek yogurt crowned with culmination and nuts; in a single day oats with berries and chia seeds; or a smoothie made with leafy veggies, almond milk, banana, and berries.

5. Snack alternatives: Keep healthful snacks on hand to control starvation amongst meals

without compromising vitamins degrees. Choose quit end result like apples or bananas; yogurt combined with fruit or granola; veggie sticks with hummus or guacamole; path combination containing nuts and dried give up end result; or whole-grain crackers with cottage cheese.

6. Guidelines for thing control: Managing portion sizes can save you immoderate weight benefit subsequently of pregnancy. Knowing the manner to visualize serving sizes may be useful For example, three to four oz Of meat can be in assessment to a deck of playing cards, whilst 1/2 a cup of cooked grains can resemble the dimensions of your clenched fist.

7. Mindful consuming: Eating slowly and consciously can enhance digestion and decrease overeating. Focus on chewing very well, casting off distractions like digital gadgets, and taking note of your frame's starvation alerts.

Chapter 9: Preparing For a Natural Birth

Understanding the Stages of Labor

As a fast-to-be mom, it's essential to understand the tiers of hard paintings so that you're better geared up to face this setting time with self guarantee and assurance. The manner of hard artwork and transport may be damaged down into 4 critical ranges – each with its particular inclinations. In this section, we will communicate those 4 levels in element and assist ease your issues approximately the device beforehand.

Stage 1: Early Labor

The first diploma of hard work is characterized via the onset of contractions. These are not to be confused with Braxton Hicks contractions, which might be usually ordinary and painless. Real contractions become ordinary, increasingly immoderate, and growing nearer collectively through the years.

During early tough paintings, your cervix begins to dilate and efface (thin out) in coaching for childbirth. This degree can take many hours or perhaps days, in particular for first-time mothers. You would possibly probable revel in moderate, cramp-like sensations as your body prepares for the following level.

During this time, it is vital to stay snug, hydrated, and nourished as an entire lot as viable. Keep your self busy at home or attempt task non-strenuous sports along side searching films or studying books that maintain you comfortable.

Stage 2: Active Labor

Active labor is marked with the aid of the use of stronger contractions that end up closer collectively (about five minutes apart) as your cervix dilates from 4-7cm. Additionally, the ones contractions ultimate longer than the ones in early tough paintings – as an awful lot as a minute or more.

This degree can be quite intense and may ultimate numerous hours. To make topics worse, a few women might possibly experience "lower once more labor" because of their little one being in a posterior function (toddler managing the mother's stomach). To contend with those excessive sensations, preserve in thoughts using rest strategies which embody deep respiratory physical video games or taking note of soothing music.

You can also strive tremendous positions like popularity, kneeling on all fours, or leaning in competition to a wall, which would possibly likely provide some remedy. Your healthcare organisation or doula (when you have one) can assist manual you via this technique and advocate most appropriate positions.

Stage three: Transition Phase

During the transition segment, your cervix dilates from 7-10cm as contractions intensify however further. This period is probably the maximum tough, with contractions being extra not unusual (each to 3 minutes), lasting up to 90 seconds.

Common symptoms at some level inside the transition segment consist of shaking, warm flashes, vomiting, and severe pressure in the lower returned and pelvic place. As tough as it might be, try to continue to be targeted and calm inside the course of this stage – use relaxation techniques found out sooner or later of prenatal commands or turn for your assist man or woman for reassurance.

Once your cervix is simply dilated at 10cm, you may skip within the path of the very last level of tough paintings – pushing.

Stage 4: Pushing and Delivery

The pushing level commonly involves additives: fetal descent and crowning of the infant's head. During fetal descent, your toddler's head drops decrease into the pelvis at the same time as you enjoy an uncontrollable urge to push.

Contractions slow down slightly about 5 mins apart but they final longer (up to 2 minutes every). Breathing deeply amongst contractions becomes critical as it allows deliver oxygen to both you and your toddler.

The crowning takes region while the most important a part of the toddler's head is seen on the vaginal organising. At this time, you will be asked to push with every contraction whilst controlling your breathing in order no longer to exhaust your self. A final few lengthy, deep pushes will signal the appearance of your little one into this global.

After turning within the child, there can be time for fast skin-to-pores and skin touch earlier than shifting on to the delivery of the placenta – a way commonly taking round half-hour. It's now time for birthday celebration and bonding together with your valuable new addition.

Understanding each degree of hard artwork can assist mitigate fear and tension surrounding the machine. Familiarize yourself with the levels, and hold in mind that your medical group is there to guide and guide you. Utilize rest and coping techniques that artwork exceptional for you, and do now not be afraid to rely on your hard paintings guide institution for help.

Creating a Birth Plan

A beginning plan serves as a manual to assist expectant moms talk their possibilities and goals for their labor, transport, and postpartum experience. It can alleviate tension via getting ready each the mom-to-be and her useful resource group for splendid conditions which can occur at some level in the transport manner. This phase will define the severa components to bear in mind whilst growing a transport plan for a herbal being pregnant.

1. Introduction: Begin growing your shipping plan through which include a short advent that consists of your call, your partner's name (if relevant), and any key touch information. This phase need to additionally include a

statement expressing your desire for a natural childbirth experience and any particular necessities or beliefs you hold spherical birthing.

2. Preferred Care Provider: If you've got got decided on a selected doula, midwife, or health practitioner to help with your herbal beginning, list their call and contact statistics on this phase. Additionally, articulate any options or expectations you could have regarding their characteristic.

3. Birth Environment: Since the surroundings substantially impacts your consolation in the route of tough work and transport, it is vital to make smooth your selections. Describe wherein you would like to offer shipping (e.G., homebirth, birthing middle, or health center) and advocate the surroundings you decide upon, which embody low lighting, calming tune, or aromatherapy.

four. Labor Support: To make sure right help inside the route of your tough paintings, virtually outline folks that may be in attendance. This may also additionally additionally encompass your associate, circle of relatives people, pals, doula, or midwife—absolutely everyone who's there to offer physical or emotional beneficial aid for the duration of the manner.

5. Techniques for Pain Management: Although herbal childbirth avoids the usage of pain medicine or epidurals, there are even though many device available to control pain efficiently. List any relaxation strategies you would love to rent all through labor (e.G., meditation or visualizations). Additionally, specify if you're open to opportunity techniques collectively with hydrotherapy (birthing pool or bath), massage, acupressure, or using a birthing ball.

6. Birth Positions: Many women find that certain positions can be greater conducive to a smoother exertions and transport. Include any preferred positions (e.G., squatting, repute, kneeling) and point out in case you

would like get right of access to to specific props or gadget.

7. Monitoring Baby's Well-being: During tough work, it's far common for healthcare carriers to display the infant's coronary coronary coronary heart rate to make certain their nicely-being. Clearly nation your alternatives concerning fetal monitoring (e.G., intermittent or non-save you), and communicate the ones alternatives collectively along with your care business employer preceding to the start.

8. Interventions and Procedures: In this segment, listing your opportunities for numerous scientific interventions. Although you are aiming for a natural childbirth enjoy, it's far critical to decide the way you would love capability interventions to be treated have to headaches rise up. Address your choices surrounding induction of tough work, membrane rupture, episiotomy, forceps delivery, vacuum extraction, and cesarean sections.

9. Postpartum Preferences: After your little one is born, there are various selections to be made approximately scientific strategies and early parenting choices. Consider the subsequent factors: instantaneous pores and skin-to-pores and skin touch among mom and little one; cord clamping opportunities; transport partner cutting the umbilical wire; management of Vitamin K injection and eye ointment; breastfeeding initiation; bathing of the toddler; vaccination schedules; and the inclusion of any cultural or spiritual rituals.

10: Flexibility Statement: Finally, well known that birthing plans can change because of surprising events. Include a announcement expressing that, in the long run, every you and your care companies are devoted to prioritizing the safety and nicely-being of every mom and toddler—however any changes required.

Creating your beginning plan is treasured in facilitating communicate collectively together together with your care employer organization whilst promoting an open communicate approximately every issue of your pregnancy journey. Providing a entire avenue map of your desires ensures that everybody concerned allows and respects your choice for a natural childbirth experience.

Natural Pain Relief Techniques

Natural being pregnant is a adventure wherein girls try to preserve their well-being and the health of their growing toddler with out relying on capsules or invasive interventions. Among the various disturbing conditions confronted in a few unspecified time within the future of being pregnant, ache manage is a crucial problem that frequently calls for attention. Here, we are capable of introduce you to herbal pain treatment strategies that may help ladies cope with pain at some point in their pregnancies.

1. Deep Breathing Exercises: One of the best but powerful techniques for coping with ache

is deep breathing. It is simple-to-observe and can create a chilled effect, predominant to decreased stress and tension. To exercise deep breathing, find out a snug function and take sluggish, deep breaths thru your nostril. Hold your breath for some seconds and exhale slowly through your mouth. Repeat the approach till you sense comfortable.

2. Prenatal Yoga: Prenatal yoga is some different natural approach to assuaging ache and pain in the course of pregnancy. It consists of stretching sporting activities, relaxation techniques, and meditation practices tailor-made for expectant mothers' desires. Regular prenatal yoga can reduce physical ache along with once more pain and joint stiffness even as fostering intellectual nicely-being at some stage in being pregnant.

3. Massage Therapy: A prenatal massage can offer massive relief from ache for pregnant ladies. Certified therapists are knowledgeable in appropriate techniques to cope with the precise desires of pregnant women gently

with out inflicting any chance to the unborn infant. Massages not handiest alleviate muscle discomfort and tension however additionally growth blood pass, contributing to ordinary properly-being.

4. Acupuncture: Acupuncture is an historic Chinese exercising that has validated promise in providing natural pain comfort in the course of pregnancy. Skilled practitioners insert thin needles into precise factors in the body to stability the body's electricity pathways or meridians, promoting recovery and decreasing soreness. While many women file exceptional results from acupuncture remedies, it is crucial to looking for advice out of your healthcare issuer before choosing this treatment.

5. Hydrotherapy: Hydrotherapy encompasses numerous water-primarily based absolutely techniques to lessen ache and soreness throughout pregnancy. Warm baths, swimming, and soothing showers can help alleviate muscle tension and offer a feel of

relaxation for pregnant ladies. Soaking in a warmth tub can art work wonders for relieving decrease lower back ache and swollen joints.

6. Aromatherapy: For centuries, crucial oils had been applied for his or her restoration homes. Aromatherapy may be practiced by using inhaling essential oils or using them topically to the pores and skin (diluted with company oil) to enjoy their healing consequences. Some oils, like lavender or chamomile, are stated to useful resource in rest and ache control inside the direction of being pregnant. However, studies the safety of specific important oils before the use of them, as a few can also moreover have terrible results in your being pregnant.

7. Heat and Cold Therapy: Basic warmth and cold remedy can beneficial useful resource in decreasing pain at some point of pregnancy. For instance, warmth compresses or heating pads might also additionally alleviate backaches or sore muscle tissues, on the

identical time as cold packs can help reduce irritation in swollen joints. Use those restoration procedures cautiously to prevent burns or frostbite – 20 mins training with breaks in among are beneficial.

eight. Meditation and Visualization: Using meditation strategies and visualization physical sports activities can assist pregnant women in dealing with tension and strain that often accompany physical pain. By accomplishing a meditative nation, you may sweep away terrible thoughts and emotions that could worsen your ache. Visualization carrying sports will let you hold a extraordinary outlook to your pregnancy adventure.

nine. Herbal Remedies: There are numerous natural herbs that declare to provide comfort from pain in the course of being pregnant, which includes ginger for morning infection or raspberry leaf tea for menstrual-like cramps. It is important to attempting to find advice from your healthcare company earlier than using any herbal treatments considering unique herbs may not be suitable all through being pregnant.

10. Support from Loved Ones: Lastly, in no manner underestimate the electricity of emotional assist from cherished ones! A compassionate partner, family member, or buddy can provide comfort that permits control ache efficaciously at a few level within the being pregnant adventure.

Chapter 10: Holistic Prenatal Care

Integrating Holistic Therapies

A herbal pregnancy emphasizes the harmony among the frame, thoughts, and spirit for the duration of this critical stage of existence. By incorporating holistic cures into your pregnancy journey, you can accumulate this stability and optimize your nicely-being. This section wills manual you thru some popular and effective holistic treatment options that can be without problem protected into your each day habitual.

1. Prenatal Yoga: Prenatal yoga is a amazing preference for strengthening the physical body and calming the mind in training for childbirth. This mild exercise focuses on stretching, deep respiration, and meditative strategies that alleviate stress and promote relaxation. Additionally, prenatal yoga can improve stamina, flexibility, and stability which can be useful all through your pregnancy Always searching for advice from an authorized teacher who is professional in

operating with pregnant women to ensure right alignment and protection.

2. Acupuncture: Acupuncture is an historical Chinese medication approach that entails placing terrific needles into specific factors at the frame to repair stability and facilitate recovery. In pregnancy, acupuncture may additionally additionally additionally help in quite a few methods which includes assuaging morning sickness, lowering pressure, coping with pain sooner or later of labor, or even turning a breech toddler. Although acupuncture is typically considered stable throughout all stages of pregnancy, typically go to a licensed practitioner to talk approximately ability risks related to fine needle placements or strategies.

three. Chiropractic Care: Chiropractic care specializes in maintaining major spinal alignment to beneficial aid general health in a few unspecified time in the future of pregnancy. By ensuring that your spine is free from misalignments or subluxations, chiropractic modifications might also moreover moreover assist reduce pain or pain related to the physical modifications of pregnancy. In addition, normal chiropractic visits have been connected to shorter tough paintings times and less interventions in the route of delivery. Be positive to visit a chiropractor who specializes in prenatal care earlier than proceeding with any treatments.

4. Herbal Remedies: Herbal treatments have been used for loads of years through numerous cultures global to manual a wholesome being pregnant. They can offer moderate, natural treatment for not unusual pregnancy-related ailments which incorporates nausea, fatigue, or insomnia. Many well-known herbs like ginger, chamomile, and raspberry leaf have an extended information of use during being pregnant. However, it's critical to go to a certified practitioner earlier than using any herbs, as some may be unstable or pose risks in your growing infant.

5. Aromatherapy: Aromatherapy makes use of crucial oils derived from flora or plants to promote emotional and physical properly-being. When properly performed, the ones oils can offer comfort from anxiety, pressure, or perhaps nausea skilled at some point of pregnancy. Lavender, frankincense, and geranium are only a few examples of safe vital oils to apply even as pregnant. Always studies the ideal dilution ratios and strategies of application for each oil and are attempting to find recommendation from an aromatherapist for similarly steering.

6. Massage Therapy: Prenatal massage therapy isn't always handiest a chilled deal with however furthermore presents numerous advantages for expectant mothers. Regular massages assist enhance blood flow, sell rest, alleviate again ache, lessen swelling within the joints or extremities and guide emotional well-being. Be tremendous to discover a certified therapist who has revel in with prenatal massage techniques.

7. Nutrition Counselling: Nutrition performs a key characteristic inside the health and nicely-being of each the mom and the developing toddler. A holistic nutritionist can provide precious steerage on consuming entire meals which can be rich in important nutrients preferred in some unspecified time in the destiny of pregnancy which includes folic acid, iron, calcium, and wholesome fats like Omega-3s. By following a tailor-made nutrient-dense weight loss program for the duration of your pregnancy journey, you can help ensure maximum effective growth and development to your toddler on the equal time as minimizing complications.

eight. Guided Meditation: Meditation is a powerful device that could assist manipulate tension or pressure at some stage in being pregnant at the same time as nurturing mindfulness and inner peace. Through guided meditation practices designed mainly for expectant mothers; you'll discover ways to cultivate deep rest techniques that can be especially useful sooner or later of difficult work and transport. Guided meditation instructions may be discovered to your community or online.

The Role of Yoga and Meditation in Natural Pregnancy

When it includes pregnancy, minimizing pressure is important for every the mother and the developing baby. One way to collect this balance is by way of manner of using incorporating yoga and meditation into each day workout routines as a part of a herbal pregnancy journey. Yoga and meditation had been practiced for loads of years as a means to promote physical, intellectual, and emotional nicely-being. In phrases of pregnancy, those ancient strategies provide a holistic approach to making sure a healthy, herbal being pregnant adventure.

Benefits of Yoga all through Pregnancy

1. Improved Physical Health: Prenatal yoga focuses on gentle stretching and strengthening bodily games that assist

decorate muscle tone, flexibility, and staying power. These sporting activities can provide alleviation from commonplace pregnancy discomforts including decrease again pain, swollen joints, or leg cramps.

2. Enhanced Mental Well-being: The exercising of yoga encourages mindfulness and strain bargain. As pregnant ladies actively work on freeing anxiety thru stretches and breathwork, they end up more able to dealing with anxiety or temper swings which can rise up because of hormonal modifications at some stage in pregnancy.

3. Increased Blood Circulation: Yoga encourages right blood motion at some point of the body. This improves oxygenation of tissues and permits reduce swelling or edema within the extremities – situations commonly professional in the route of being pregnant.

four. Reduced Risk of Gestational Diabetes: Regular prenatal yoga exercise must potentially reduce the risk of growing gestational diabetes due to its awesome impact on blood glucose tiers.

5. Labor Preparation: The deep respiratory techniques applied in yoga can contribute to natural childbirth with the useful resource of supporting girls bring together their stamina for labor and education them to attention their strength for the duration of contractions. Flexibility received from prenatal yoga can also facilitate childbirth with the useful resource of making an allowance for cushty positioning throughout labor.

Benefits of Meditation at some point of Pregnancy

1. Lower Stress Levels: Meditation permits pregnant women to cultivate a enjoy of calmness and peace. By developing a snug highbrow state, meditation can assist reduce strain hormones, in the long run selling the well-being of every the mother and her infant.

2. Improved Sleep: The relaxation acquired thru meditation will have a immoderate fine impact on sleep patterns, this is critical for everyday fitness and thoughts development within the route of being pregnant.

3. Enhanced Bonding: Meditation can provide a quiet vicinity for expectant moms to music into their our bodies and be part of more deeply with their unborn toddlers. Focusing at the baby's heartbeat, movements, or possibly visualizing the infant within the womb can enhance the maternal bond.

4. Preparation for Childbirth: Meditation teaches strategies that may be used in the course of hard work for pain control and maintaining a targeted, comfortable nation of mind.

The key to reaping the blessings of yoga and meditation at some point of being pregnant lies in consistency – making the ones practices part of your every day normal is critical. Here are some tips to help you get started out:

1. Consult with a expert: It is critical to go to your healthcare company or a licensed prenatal yoga trainer before beginning any new exercising habitual at some point of being pregnant.

2. Listen in your body: Pregnancy is not the time to push your body past its limits. Practice mild, gradual movements that specialize in connecting along with your breath even as maintaining mindfulness and keeping off forceful practices like strength yoga.

3. Practice with steerage: If you're new to yoga or meditation, keep in mind joining a prenatal yoga beauty especially designed for expectant moms or following guided meditations created for being pregnant.

four. Create a snug area: Set up a cushty region in your house committed to operating in the direction of yoga and meditation – this can make it an awful lot much less complicated to include those practices into your each day every day.

5. Be steady: Aim for as a minimum 10-15 minutes of every day workout – even small amounts of consistent exercising can bring about large benefits over the years.

Holistic Approaches to Common Pregnancy Discomforts

Below are a number of the holistic strategies that can help alleviate common being pregnant discomforts. With a focus on natural remedies and treatment plans, allows dive into the diverse global of holistic care throughout being pregnant.

1. Morning Sickness: Morning sickness is one of the most common being pregnant discomforts, affecting a majority of pregnant girls. While there isn't a one-duration-suits-all therapy for morning sickness, the following holistic remedies can help alleviate symptoms and signs and symptoms and signs and symptoms:

a) Ginger: Ginger has prolonged been used to address nausea and vomiting associated with morning contamination. You can strive ginger tablets, ginger tea, or possibly which incorporates sparkling ginger to your meals.

b) Vitamin B6: Studies have demonstrated that taking nutrients B6 dietary nutritional dietary supplements can lessen nausea and vomiting in the course of being pregnant. Consult collectively together with your healthcare company in advance than taking any dietary supplements.

c) Acupressure: Applying pressure to particular factors at the frame can help lessen nausea. One such detail is the P6 factor on the wrist, known as Nei Guan. Acupressure wristbands are widely to be had and designed to intention this unique component.

2. Lower Back Pain: Lower again pain is any other ache skilled with the useful resource of maximum pregnant girls due to hormonal adjustments and elevated weight advantage. Holistic techniques to alleviate lower returned pain encompass:

a) Prenatal Yoga: Prenatal yoga focuses on poses that beautify your center muscle tissue on the equal time as improving flexibility and stability, that allows you to in the long run assist ease your lower returned pain.

b) Chiropractic Care: A licensed chiropractor can assist realign your spine and pelvis, reducing pressure on your lower returned and lowering pain.

c) Massage: A professional prenatal rub down can help relieve muscle anxiety and improve pass, as a end result decreasing lower again pain.

3. Constipation: Hormones released ultimately of being pregnant generally tend to gradual down the digestive machine, inflicting constipation in many pregnant ladies. To keep away from constipation during pregnancy, attempt the following holistic remedies:

a) High-Fiber Diet: Include extra immoderate-fiber elements collectively with entire grains, give up quit result, and vegetables on your diet regime to help make certain regular bowel moves.

b) Staying Hydrated: Drinking enough water is critical for correct digestion and stopping constipation.

c) Regular Exercise: Light to moderate physical hobby which encompass strolling or swimming can help stimulate bowel moves and relieve constipation.

4. Swelling and Edema: Swelling can arise because of accelerated blood amount and fluid retention during being pregnant. While it is also harmless, excessive swelling may additionally reason ache. To reduce swelling truly, attempt the following holistic strategies:

a) Elevation: Elevate your legs above coronary heart diploma each time feasible to lower swelling.

b) Compression Socks: Wearing compression socks can assist improve bypass and decrease infection on your decrease limbs.

c) Magnesium Supplements: Some studies have suggested that taking magnesium nutritional dietary supplements may help alleviate edema in pregnant girls. However, continuously speak over along with your healthcare company in advance than taking dietary supplements.

5. Fatigue: Fatigue is another common pregnancy discomfort, specifically inside the first trimester. Holistic methods to fight fatigue encompass:

a) Prioritizing Rest: Make positive you get sufficient sleep at night time and take naps even as wanted.

b) Balanced Diet: A properly-balanced, nutrient-dense food regimen can help provide strength to combat fatigue throughout being pregnant.

c) Moderate Exercise: Light exercise which incorporates on foot or stretching can help growth energy tiers while you're feeling fatigued.

6. Heartburn: Heartburn can also get up due to hormonal changes and a developing uterus that places stress at the belly for the duration of being pregnant. To alleviate heartburn sincerely, keep in mind these holistic treatments:

a) Avoiding Trigger Foods: Steering easy of spicy, fatty, or acidic food can reduce heartburn occurrences.

b) Eating Small Meals Frequently: Consuming smaller meals at some point of the day in choice to 3 big ones can restrict heartburn signs and symptoms and symptoms and signs.

c) Sleeping with an Elevated Upper Body: Propping up your top frame at the identical time as slumbering can help save you belly acid from flowing lower back into the esophagus.

Chapter 11: A Natural Approach to Nutrition

Building a Nutrient-Dense Diet

During being pregnant, it's essential for mothers to prioritize their health and well being. Building a nutrient-dense diet guarantees which you and your baby receive all of the nutrients, minerals, and macronutrients wanted for predominant growth and improvement. Let us communicate critical vitamins, find out particular food assets, and offer practical guidelines to make sure a balanced weight loss plan at some point of being pregnant.

1. Essential Nutrients for Pregnancy: A nutrient-dense healthy eating plan includes numerous essential nutrients that assist your body's wishes in a few unspecified times in the destiny of being pregnant. Here is a listing of essential vitamins to embody in your meal plan:

a) Folic Acid: Folic acid is vital for the healthy improvement of your infant's neural tube and the formation of pink blood cells. Consider consuming leafy veggies, legumes, citrus surrender result, fortified cereals, or prenatal dietary supplements to fulfill the endorsed every day intake.

b) Iron: Iron allows oxygen shipping inside the blood and the producing of hemoglobin. Good belongings encompass lean meat, chicken, fish, fortified cereals, legumes, tofu, and inexperienced greens.

c) Calcium: Calcium is essential for robust bones and teeth in each mother and infant. It moreover aids in nerve function and muscle contractions. Opt for dairy products, leafy vegetables, almonds, broccoli, or calcium-fortified meals-drinks.

d) Vitamin D: Vitamin D guarantees right bone improvement via supporting your frame soak up calcium efficiently. Sources include fatty fish, daylight hour's publicity (with caution), egg yolks, fortified milk or orange juice.

e) Omega-three Fatty Acids: Omega-three fatty acids play an vital role in fetal mind improvement. Incorporate salmon, mackerel, herring, walnuts or chia seeds into your diet regime regularly.

f) Protein: Proteins are constructing blocks for cells in each mom and little one; select lean meats, fish, beans, legumes, nuts or seeds to satisfy you're every day requirement.

g) Fiber: Fiber prevents constipation and permits regulate blood sugar degrees inside the path of pregnancy. Consume complete grains, veggies, cease end result, and legumes to make sure right daily intake.

2. Navigating Nutrient-Dense Food: In addition to essential vitamins, it's miles useful to understand the one of kind meals companies and their respective benefits.

a) Fruits: Fruits are complete of nutrients, minerals, and antioxidants. They additionally provide hydration and offer natural sweetness for a wholesome pregnancy weight loss plan.

b) Vegetables: Vegetables supply critical nutrients like fiber, folate, potassium, and severa nutrients. Aim to eat a colorful array of vegetables each day as a part of your nutrient-dense weight loss plan.

c) Grains: Whole grains offer fiber and B-vitamins that resource in power manufacturing. Select complete-wheat bread, pasta, brown rice or quinoa over sensitive grains for optimum nutrition.

d) Protein: A protein-rich eating regimen permits fetal growth and development on the identical time as maintaining mother's muscle tissue. Rotate amongst animal and plant-primarily based proteins for variety and balanced nutrients.

e) Dairy: Calcium-rich dairy merchandise help bring together strong bones on your child. Choose low-fats milk, yogurt, or cheese for high-quality intake without greater saturated fats.

3. Practical Tips for Building a Nutrient-Dense Diet

a) Meal Planning: Create a weekly meal plan that includes severa food corporations, and account on your day by day nutrient dreams. Variety ensures most suitable nutrients intake even as maintaining food exciting.

b) Snacking Smartly: Choose wholesome snacks like yogurt with fruit, nuts with dried fruit or carrot sticks with hummus to satisfy starvation among food without sacrificing nutrients.

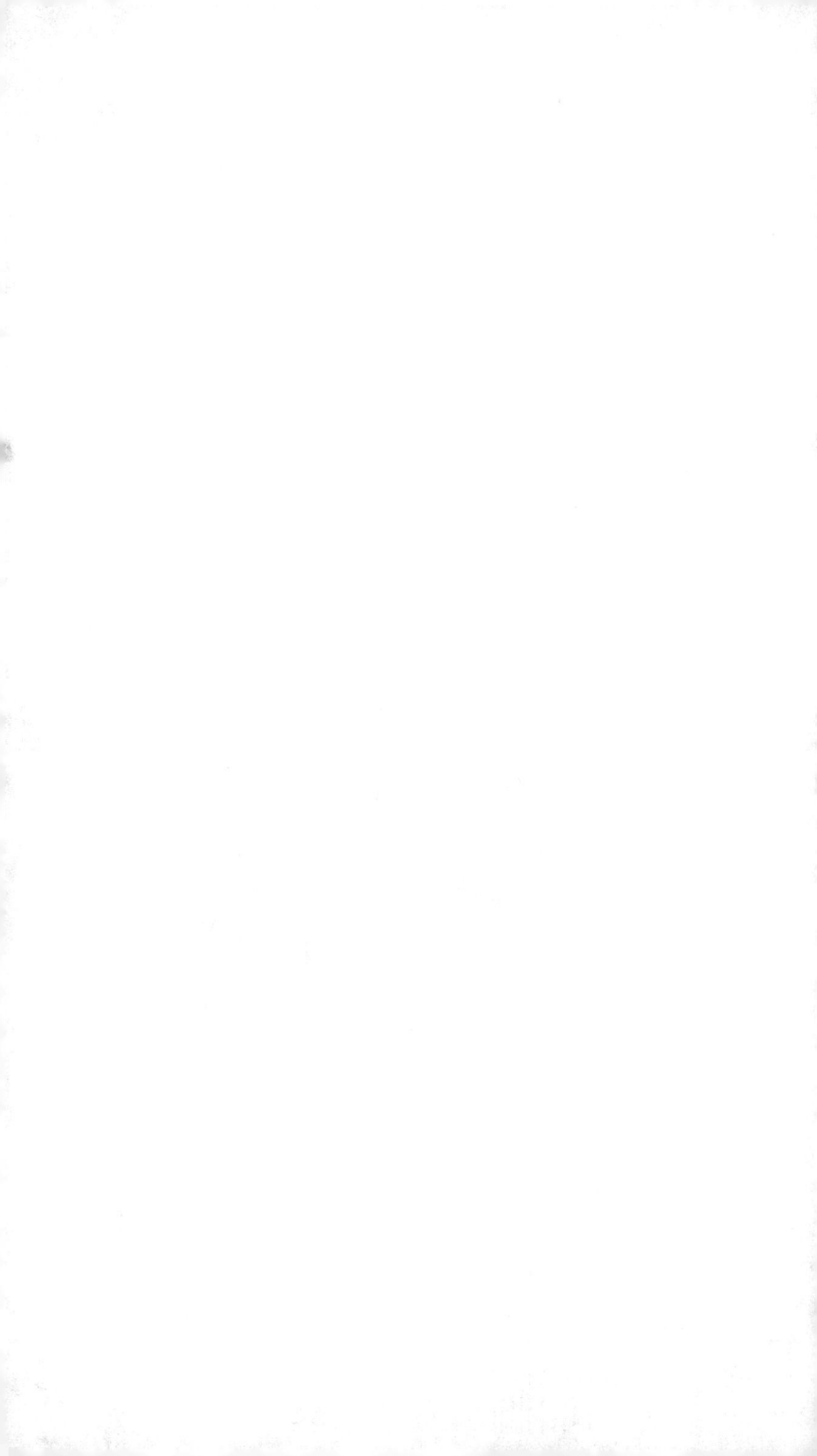

www.ingramcontent.com/pod-product-compliance
Lightning Source LLC
Chambersburg PA
CBHW051727020426
42333CB00014B/1194